Challenges in Pancreatic Cancer

Edited by Mila Dimitrova Kovacheva-Slavova and Borislav Georgiev Vladimirov

Published in London, United Kingdom

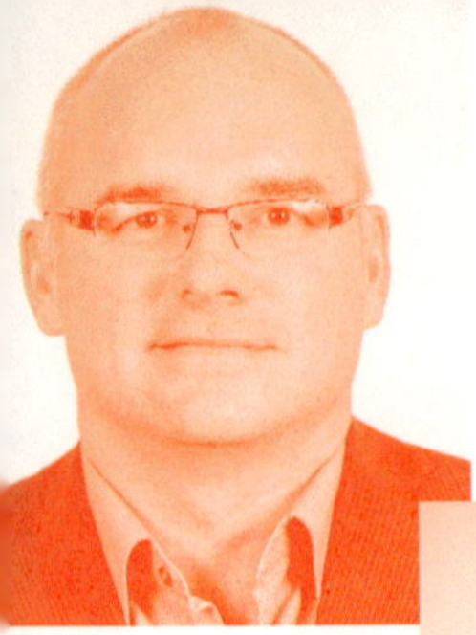
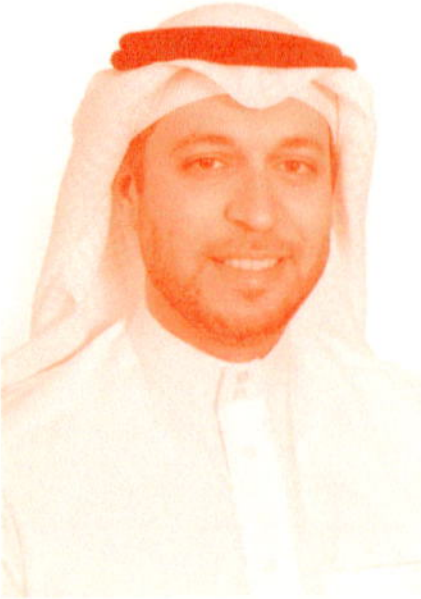
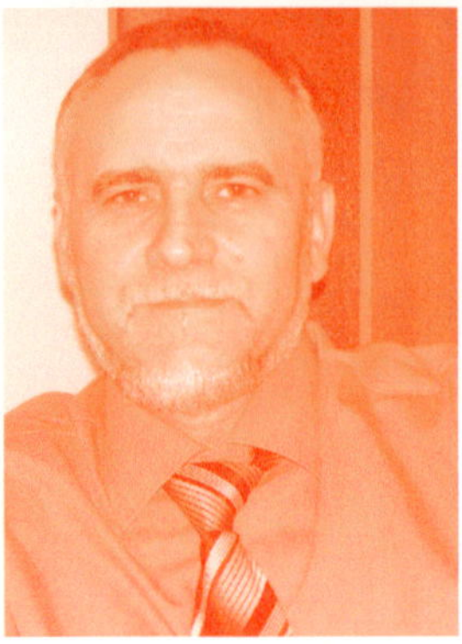
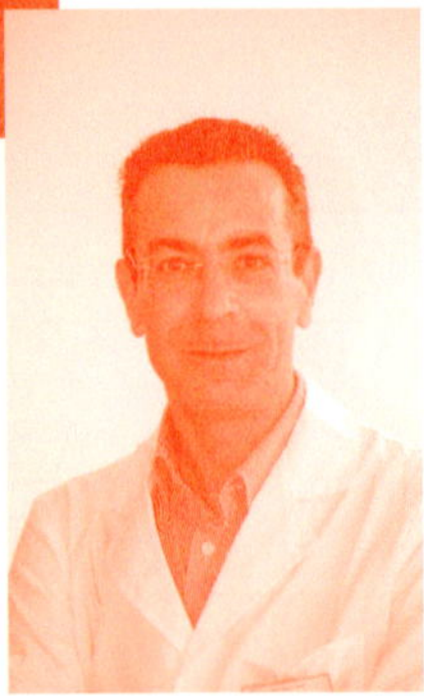
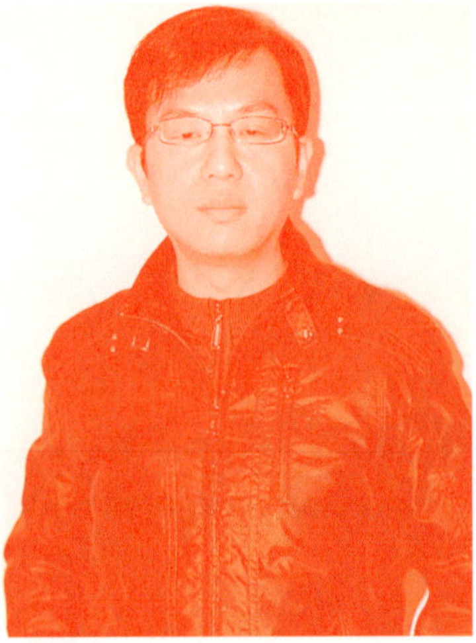
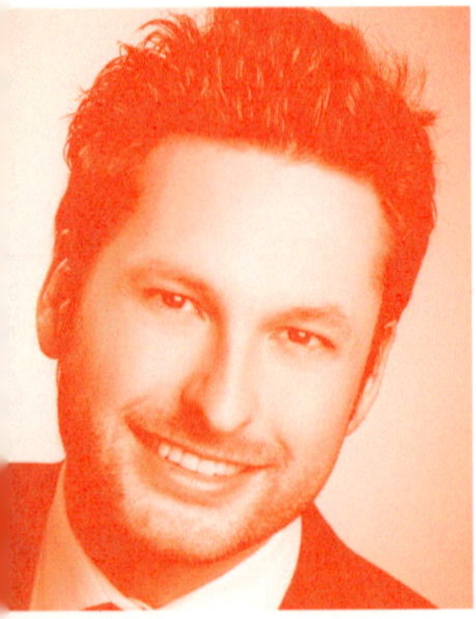
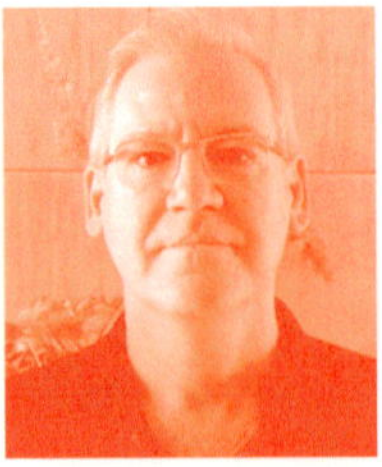

IntechOpen

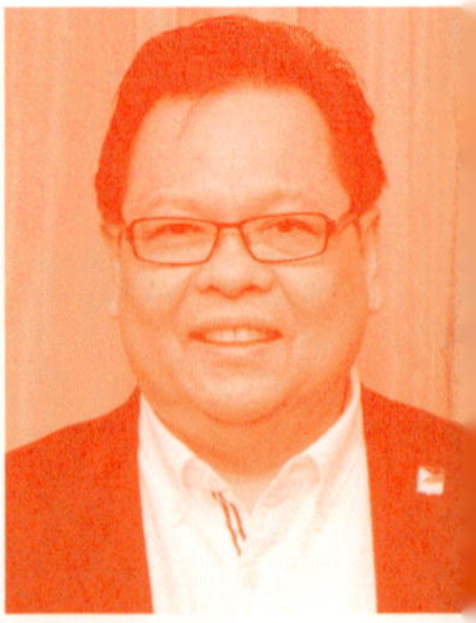
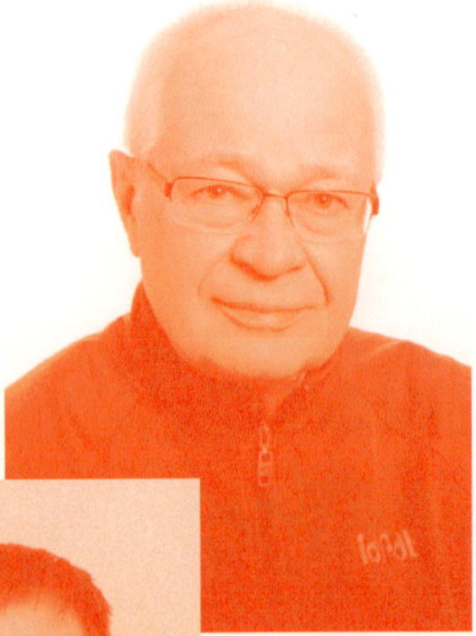
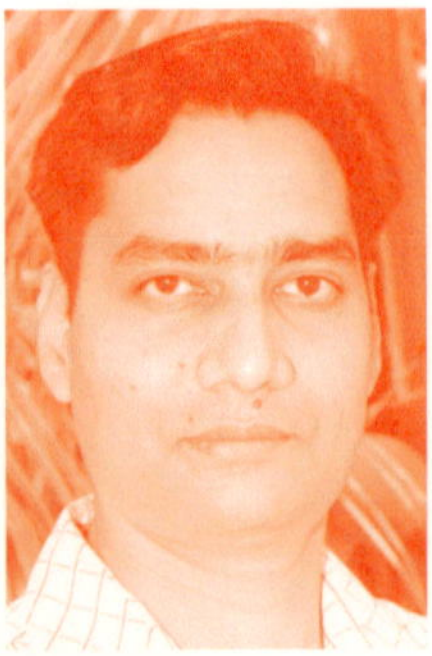
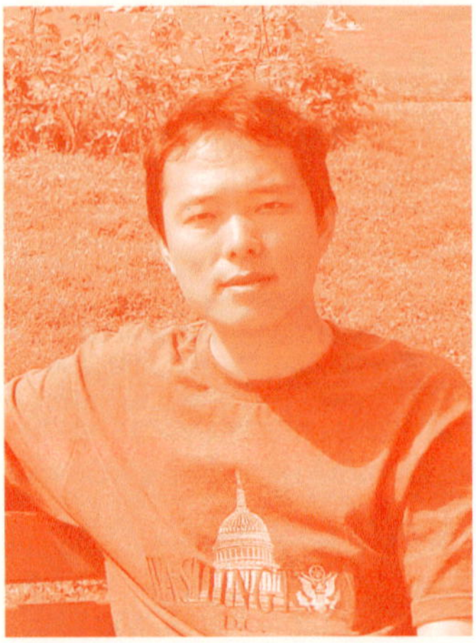
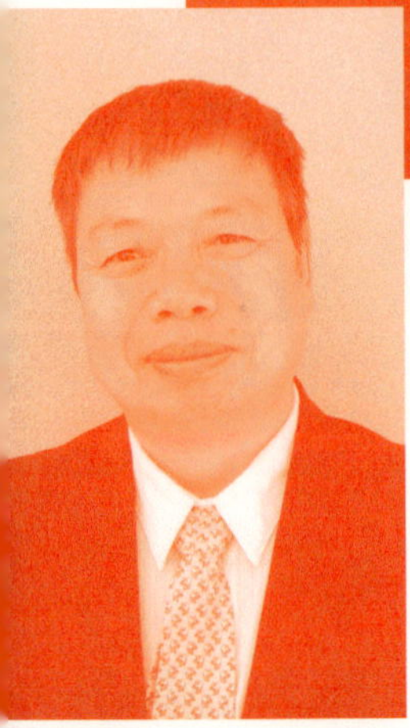
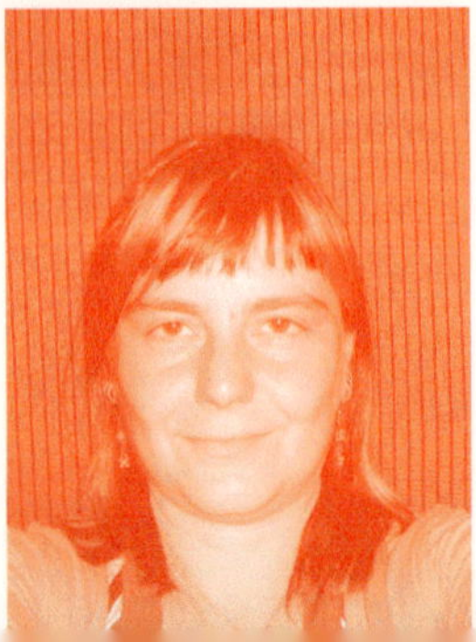

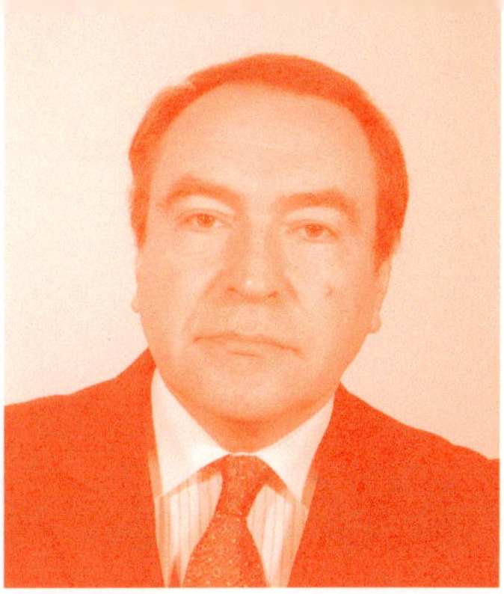
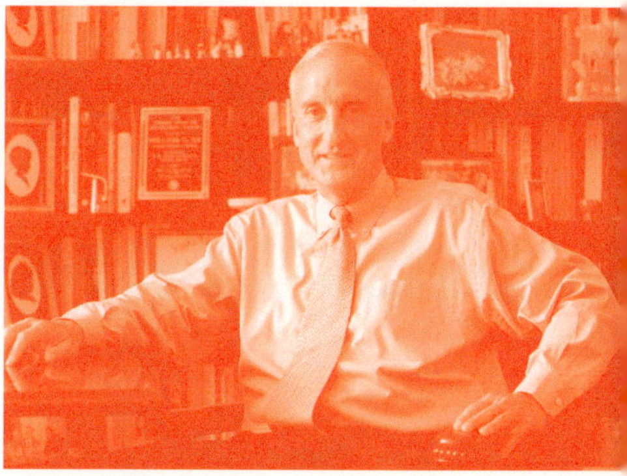
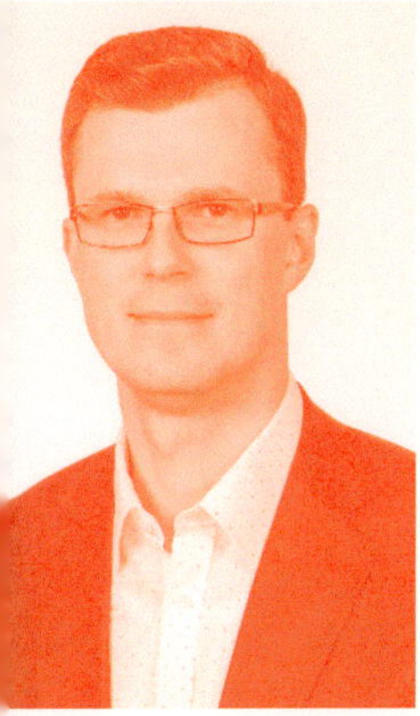
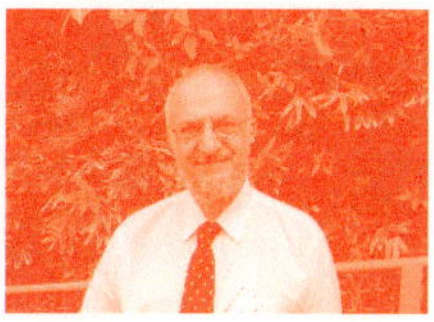
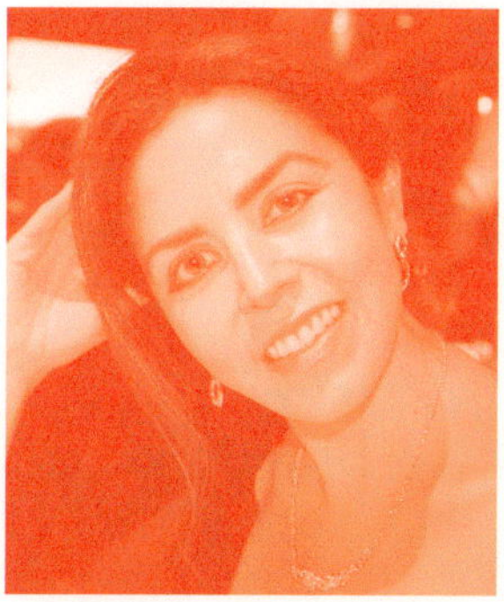

Supporting open minds since 2005

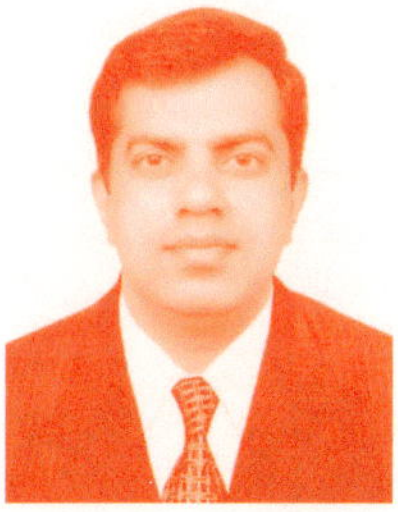
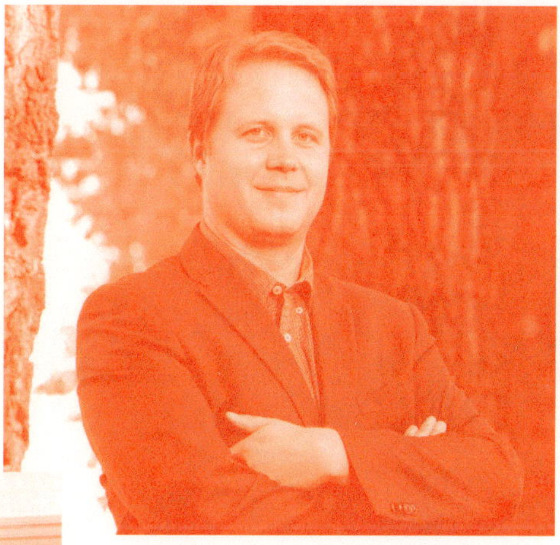
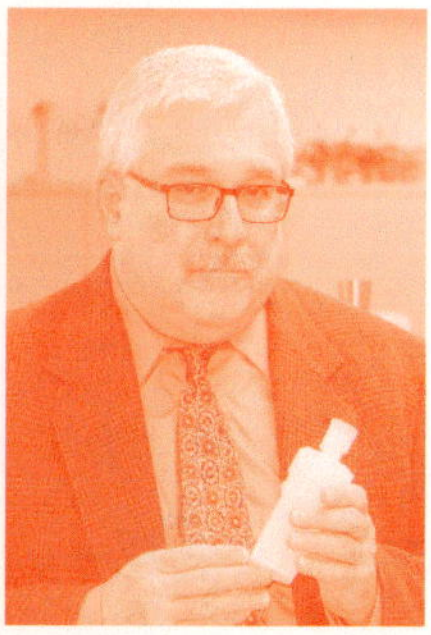
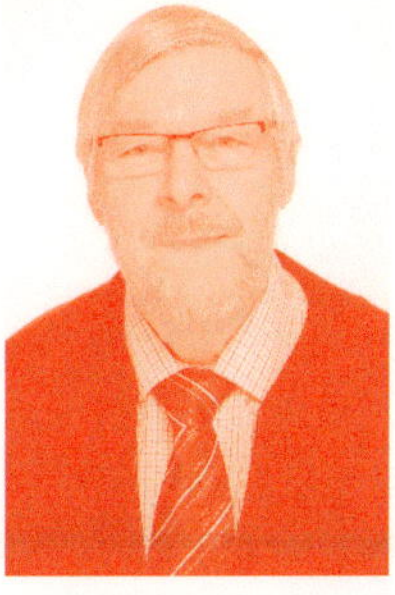
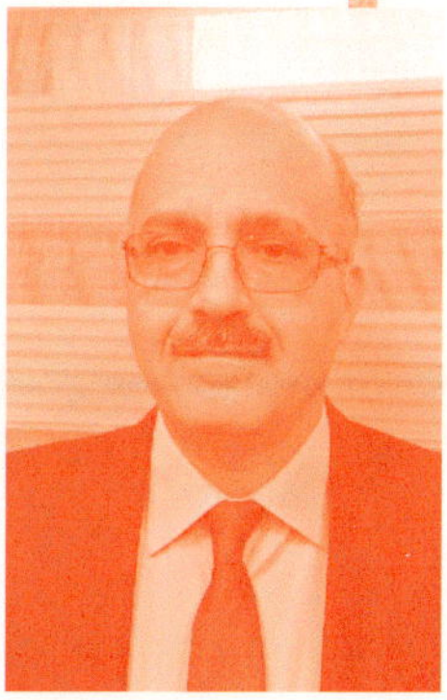
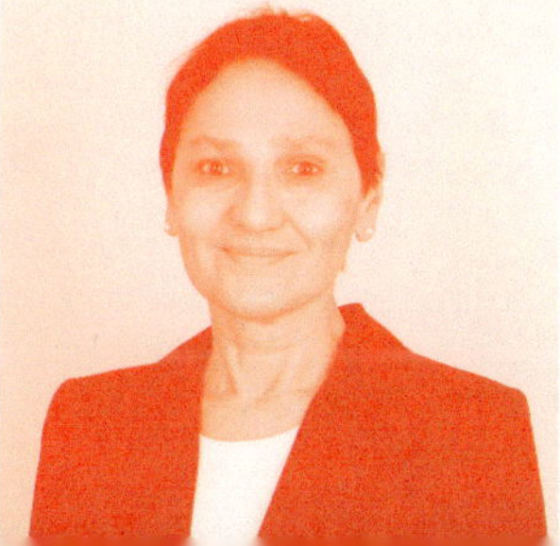
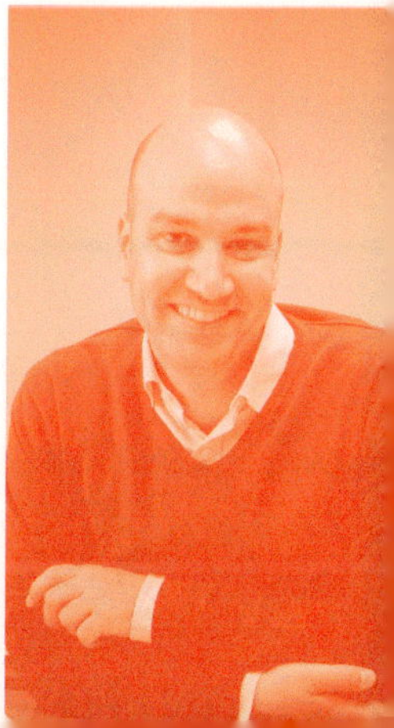

Challenges in Pancreatic Cancer
http://dx.doi.org/10.5772/intechopen.87597
Edited by Mila Dimitrova Kovacheva-Slavova and Borislav Georgiev Vladimirov

Contributors
Haitao Zhu, Xiaojie Cai, Yanfang Liu, Jie Gao, Qiulian Ma, Dongqing Wang, Ming Wang, Miguel Ángel Vargas Mejía, Paola Briseño Díaz, Pedro Cruz-Nova, Martiniano Bello Ramirez, Jose Correa Basurto, Dora Emma Velez-Uriza, Ma del Rocio Thompson Bonilla, Rosaura Hernadez-Rivas, Christian Caglevic, Mauricio Mahave, Cristobal Sanhueza, Luis Ubillos, Benjamin Eigl, Andreas Andreou, Matthias Peterhans, Stefan Weber, Beat Gloor, Neha Sharma, Deepti Sharma, Mila Kovacheva-Slavova, Borislav Vladimirov, Aihua Gong

First published in London, United Kingdom, 2021 by IntechOpen
IntechOpen is the global imprint of INTECHOPEN LIMITED, registered in England and Wales, registration number: 11086078, 5 Princes Gate Court, London, SW7 2QJ, United Kingdom
Printed in Croatia

British Library Cataloguing-in-Publication Data
A catalogue record for this book is available from the British Library

Additional hard and PDF copies can be obtained from orders@intechopen.com

Challenges in Pancreatic Cancer
Edited by Mila Dimitrova Kovacheva-Slavova and Borislav Georgiev Vladimirov
p. cm.
Print ISBN 978-1-83962-958-7
Online ISBN 978-1-83962-959-4
eBook (PDF) ISBN 978-1-83962-960-0

For EU product safety concerns:
IN TECH d.o.o., Prolaz Marije Krucifikse Kozulić 3, 51000 Rijeka, Croatia, info@intechopen.com or visit our website at intechopen.com.

Meet the editors

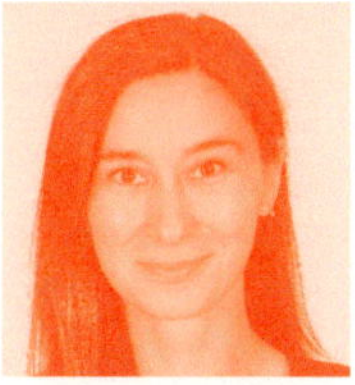

Dr. Mila Kovacheva-Slavova graduated from Medical University, Sofia, Bulgaria, where she obtained her Ph.D. in the area of pancreatic disorders. She is an assistant professor in the Department of Gastroenterology, Medical University, Sofia, and is an active member in many national and international research projects. Dr. Kovacheva-Slavova's research interests include diagnosis, therapy, and follow-up of pancreatic diseases, gastrointestinal autoimmune diseases, tumors of the digestive system, and *Helicobacter pylori* infection. Her scientific work has been presented at numerous meetings and awarded at prestigious congresses in Europe, the United States, and South America.

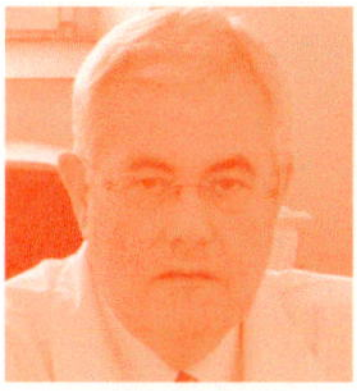

Prof. Vladimirov is head of the Department of Gastroenterology, Medical University, Sofia, Bulgaria, where he obtained his Ph.D. in the area of endoscopy treatment of bile ducts and pancreatic diseases. His main research interests are gastrointestinal diagnostic and therapeutic endoscopy, peptic diseases, Helicobacter pylori infection, and tumors of the digestive system. His main activities include digestive endoscopy, education (pre- and post-graduate), and clinical research. Dr. Vladimirov is a coordinator of many national and international projects. He has published more than 200 articles in Bulgarian and international medical journals. Dr. Vladimirov is a member of several Bulgarian and European scientific societies.

Contents

Preface

Pancreatic cancer is one of the most lethal solid organ tumors with a poor five-year survival rate despite current oncological advances. Pancreatic cancer may arise from the exocrine part of the gland (adenocarcinomas) or from the endocrine pancreas (pancreatic neuroendocrine tumors). The early and proper diagnosis of pancreatic cancer is of great importance for the improvement of the overall prognosis. Symptoms such as progressive weight loss, anorexia, abdominal pain, and jaundice appear late in the disease course and are nonspecific. Recent advances in and increasing sensitivity of diagnostic techniques such as multi-detector row computed tomography, magnetic resonance imaging, positron emission tomography, and endoscopic ultrasound are promising for early detection, staging, and differentiation of pancreatic cancer from other pancreatic diseases. Prognosis and treatment depend on the stage of pancreatic cancer; treatment strategies include surgery, ablation, chemotherapy, radiation therapy, and palliative care. There is increasing interest in the tumor microenvironment and the potential of treatment options. This book includes six chapters covering the current challenges and states of pancreatic cancer and pancreatic neuroendocrine tumors, including information on diagnostic tools, treatment strategies, and mechanisms of pancreatic cancer therapy resistance. The book is an ideal reference for a wide audience interested in the different fields of pancreatology.

For their frankness and diligence in reviewing the proposed chapters, we would like to thank all the authors who have contributed to this book. We have incorporated many of their recommendations and the book is much improved as a consequence.

Special thanks go to the staff at IntechOpen, especially Author Service Managers Dolores Kuzelj, Rebekah Pribetic, and Nina Kalinic Babic, and Commissioning Editor Lucija Tomicic-Dromgool, for their dedicated support in the reviewing process and their suggestions for further improvements.

Mila Dimitrova Kovacheva-Slavova
and Borislav Georgiev Vladimirov
Department of Gastroenterology,
University Hospital "Tsaritsa Ioanna-ISUL",
Medical University of Sofia,
Sofia, Bulgaria

Chapter 1

Introductory Chapter: Pancreatic Cancer

Mila Dimitrova Kovacheva-Slavova
and Borislav Georgiev Vladimirov

1. Introduction

Pancreatic cancer remains one of the most lethal solid organ tumors with a poor 5-year survival rate despite current oncological advances. The poor prognosis is related mostly to the late clinical manifestation. Patients usually are diagnosed in an unresectable stage when metastases are present [1]. 85% of the cases of pancreatic cancer are adenocarcinomas [2]. Pancreatic neuroendocrine tumors (NETs) are rare tumors with highly variable behaviors from nearly benign to extremely aggressive [3]. The early and proper diagnosis of pancreatic cancer is of a great importance for the improvement of the ovSerall prognosis. Symptoms are nonspecific and include progressive weight loss, anorexia, abdominal pain and jaundice. The recent advances and increasing sensitivity of the diagnostic techniques such as multi-detector-row computed tomography (MDCT), magnetic resonance imaging (MRI), positron emission tomography (PET) CT and endoscopic ultrasound (EUS) are promising for the early pancreatic cancer detection, staging and differentiation from other pancreatic diseases [4]. The resectability of the tumor depends on the possible infiltration of vessels and lymph nodes as well as distant metastases. The pancreastic cancer is resectable, borderline resectable, locally advanced or metastatic. Prognosis and treatment depend on the stage of pancreatic cancer as treatment strategies include surgery, ablation, chemotherapy, radiation therapy, and palliative care [5].

2. Challenging the pancreatic cancer

Less than 20% of the patients with pancreatic cancer are diagnosed in an early resectable stage, achieving a negative resection margin (R0) and a significant survival improvement [5, 6]. An adjuvant chemotherapy is mostly recommended after pancreatic resection [5]. A recent metaanalysis highlights the beneficial effect of neoadjuvant therapy in borderline and locally advanced pancreatic tumors, associated with a decreased tumor-stage, higher rates of R0-resections, lower rates of lymphnode invasion, decreased frequency of lymphatic vessel and perineural invasion [7]. After biopsy confirmation, chemotherapy is the treatment of choice for unresectable pancreatic cancer. Different regiments such as gemcitabine / erlotinib, FOLFIRINOX, gemcitabine /NAB-paclitaxel, gemcitabine/capecitabine, and capecitabine/oxaliplatin (XELOX) are recommended according to the patient's performance status [8]. Palliative care relieves symptoms and ensures optimal quality of life [5]. According to the complications of pancreatic cancer, patients might need endoscopic placement of stents for treating biliary obstruction, pancreatic enzyme replacement therapy for pancreatic exocrine insufficiency, insulin for

IntechOpen

treating diabetes mellitus, gastrojejunostomy, enteral stent or PEG tube in case of gastric outlet obstruction, as well as pain management and nutritive support [8–11]. Increasing is the interest on the tumor microenvironment and the arising potential future treatment option. Current clinical trials investigate promising treatment strategies for advanced pancreatic cancer such as stroma modifying drugs, platinum chemotherapy, RAS-directed therapies, immunotherapy with pembrolizumab, immune checkpoint inhibitor combinations or natural killer cells [12–14].

Author details

Mila Dimitrova Kovacheva-Slavova* and Borislav Georgiev Vladimirov
Department of Gastroenterology, University Hospital "Tsaritsa Ioanna-ISUL", Medical University of Sofia, Sofia, Bulgaria

*Address all correspondence to: kovacheva_mila@abv.bg

References

[1] Kamisawa T., Wood L.D., Itoi T., Takaori K. Pancreatic cancer. Lancet. 2016;388:73-85. doi: 10.1016/S0140-6736(16)00141-0.

[2] Siegel RL, Miller KD, Jemal A: Cancer statistics, 2015. CA Cancer J Clin 2015;65:5-29.

[3] Ro, C., Chai, W., Yu, V. E., & Yu, R. (2013). Pancreatic neuroendocrine tumors: Biology, diagnosis,and treatment. Chinese journal of cancer, *32*(6), 312-324. https://doi.org/10.5732/cjc.012.10295

[4] Miura, F., Takada, T., Amano, H., Yoshida, M., Furui, S., & Takeshita, K. (2006). Diagnosis of pancreatic cancer. HPB : the official journal of the International Hepato Pancreato Biliary Association, *8*(5), 337-342. https://doi.org/10.1080/13651820500540949

[5] Brunner, M., Wu, Z., Krautz, C., Pilarsky, C., Grützmann, R., & Weber, G. F. (2019). Current clinical strategies of pancreatic Cancer treatment and open molecular questions. International journal of molecular sciences, *20*(18), 4543. https://doi.org/10.3390/ijms20184543

[6] Kamisawa T., Wood L.D., Itoi T., Takaori K. Pancreatic cancer. Lancet. 2016;388:73-85. doi: 10.1016/S0140-6736(16)00141-0.

[7] Schorn S, Demir IE, Reyes CM, Saricaoglu C, Samm N, Schirren R, Tieftrunk E, Hartmann D, Friess H, Ceyhan GO. The impact of neoadjuvant therapy on the histopathological features of pancreatic ductal adenocarcinoma - a systematic review and meta-analysis. Cancer Treat Rev. 2017 Apr;55:96-106. doi: 10.1016/j.ctrv.2017.03.003. Epub 2017 Mar 14. PMID: 28342938.

[8] Qiubo Zhang, Linjuan Zeng, Yinting Chen, Guoda Lian, Chenchen Qian, Shaojie Chen, Jiajia Li, Kaihong Huang, "Pancreatic Cancer epidemiology, detection, and management", *Gastroenterology Research and Practice*, Vol. 2016, Article ID 8962321, 10 Pages, 2016. https://doi.org/10.1155/2016/8962321

[9] Glazer E.S., Hornbrook M.C., Krouse R.S. A meta-analysis of randomized trials: Immediate stent placement vs. surgical bypass in the palliative management of malignant biliary obstruction. J. Pain Symptom Manag. 2014;47:307-314. doi: 10.1016/j.jpainsymman.2013.03.013.

[10] Jeurnink S.M., Van Eijck C.H., Steyerberg E.W., Kuipers E.J., Siersema P.D. Stent versus gastrojejunostomy for the palliation of gastric outlet obstruction: A systematic review. BMC Gastroenterol. 2007;7:18. doi: 10.1186/1471-230X-7-18.

[11] Zhong W., Yu Z., Zeng J.X., Lin Y., Yu T., Min X.H., Yuan Y.H., Chen Q.K. Celiac plexus block for treatment of pain associated with pancreatic cancer: A meta-analysis. Pain Pract. 2014;14:43-51. doi: 10.1111/papr.12083.

[12] Network CGAR Integrated genomic characterization of pancreatic ductal adenocarcinoma. Cancer Cell. 2017;32:185-203. doi: 10.1016/j.ccell.2017.07.007.

[13] Waddell N., Pajic M., Patch A.-M., Chang D.K., Kassahn K.S., Bailey P., Johns A.L., Miller D.K., Nones K., Quek K., et al. Whole genomes redefine the mutational landscape of pancreatic cancer. Nature. 2015;518:495-501. doi: 10.1038/nature14169.

[14] Hessmann E., Johnsen S.A., Siveke J.T., Ellenrieder V. Epigenetic treatment of pancreatic cancer: Is there a therapeutic perspective on the horizon? Gut. 2017;66:168-179. doi: 10.1136/gutjnl-2016-312539.

Chapter 2

Advance in Pancreatic Cancer Diagnosis and Therapy

Xiaojie Cai, Jie Gao, Yanfang Liu, Ming Wang, Qiulian Ma, Aihua Gong, Dongqing Wang and Haitao Zhu

Abstract

Pancreatic carcinoma is the fourth leading cause of cancer death in the word wild. Although the advance in treatment this disease, the 5-years survival rate is still rather low. In the recent year, many new therapy and treatment avenues have been developed for pancreatic cancer. In this chapter, we mainly focus on the following aspect: 1) the treatment modality in pancreatic cancer, including chemotherapy, radiotherapy, and immunotherapy; 2) the mechanism of pancreatic cancer treatment resistance, especially in cancer stem cells and tumor microenvironment; 3) the diagnosis tools in pancreatic cancer, including serum markers, imaging methods and endoscopic ultrasonography. Novel molecular probes based on the nanotechnology in the diagnosis of pancreatic cancer are also discussed.

Keywords: pancreatic carcinoma, immunotherapy, cancer stem cell, tumor microenvironment, nano-medicine

1. Introduction

Pancreatic cancer is currently the fourth leading cause of cancer-related death and is predicted to be the most common cause of cancer mortality by 2030 [1]. Despite advances in the treatment of pancreatic cancer, prognosis remains extremely poor with 5-year survival of only 8% [2]. The low survival rate is attributed to several factors, such as asymptomatic until the disease develops to an advanced stage, early and extensive metastasis, and high resistance to treatment. Therefore, precision diagnosis and effective treatment is a critical clinical issue.

Currently, commonly employed treatments for pancreatic cancer include surgery, chemotherapy, and radiation therapy. Surgical resection is regarded as the only treatment for curing pancreatic cancer. However, only 15% of pancreatic cancer patients present with disease that are resectable upfront. Chemotherapy is the mainstream treatment for local, advanced and metastatic pancreatic cancer [3]. Among the traditional treatment, chemotherapy is the most advanced modality, especially the target therapy. The role of radiotherapy in pancreatic cancer is still controversial. Although the clinical trial results were disappointing, immunotherapy is the still greatly investigated approaches in pancreatic cancer. The deeper investigation of treatment resistance mechanism and novelty modality development is urgently needed.

2. Treatment modality of pancreatic cancer

At present, commonly employed treatment for pancreatic cancer include surgery, chemotherapy, and radiotherapy. The treatment options depend on the stage of pancreatic cancer. Some emerging therapeutic technologies have yet to mature, such as molecular targeted therapy and immunotherapy.

2.1 Surgical therapy

Surgical resection is regarded as the only treatment for cure and can result in significantly longer survival of pancreatic cancer. According to the diseased localization and extension, pancreatic cancer is divided into resectable, borderline resectable, or locally advanced. Resectable cases account for 15% of pancreatic cancer patients and this subpopulation is the only potential for cure. However, 5-year survival is at best 20–25%. Borderline resectable cases account for another 5–10%. For some patients with early recurrence or not have the complications of aggressive disease and latent metastasis, neoadjuvant therapy is one alternative measures to reduce the tumor burden and obtain better local control. The proper sequence of surgical therapy and neoadjuvant therapy is the determine factor. Delivering full-dose chemotherapy preoperative therapy may be more effective than postoperative therapy because the resected tumor bed is associated with poor drug delivery. In patients with borderline resectable pancreatic cancer after effective neoadjuvant therapies, the possibility for an R0 resection is higher, and survival of patients who underwent surgical resection is better than that of those who did not [4]. Approximately 30–40% of patients have locally advanced unresectable pancreatic cancer (LAPC) in which tumor is involvement of neighboring blood vessels [5].

2.2 Chemotherapy

Chemotherapy is the mainstay treatment for advanced and metastatic pancreatic cancer. Fluorouracil and gemcitabine are the first line chemotherapy drugs. However, their clinic effective is still disappointing. In recent years, the National Comprehensive Cancer Network (NCCN) guidelines have recommended two options: one is the FOLFIRINOX regimen of four drug combination (fluorouracil + calcium folate + oxaliplatin + irinotecan), another is the AG regimen of a combination of paclitaxel and gemcitabine [6]. Although the four-drug combination scheme is effective to some extent, its toxicity and side effects are great. Considering the physical strength score of some patients, the application of this scheme is limited. The albumin paclitaxel regimen is relatively safe and has fewer adverse reactions. More and more researches recommend this regimen as the first-line treatment of pancreatic cancer in the future. The following subsets are specially suitable for the albumin paclitaxel treatment, such as neoadjuvant and salvage chemotherapy patients, postoperative adjuvant chemotherapy patients, and advanced chemotherapy patients [7].

2.3 Radiotherapy

Radiotherapy is always used as a curative treatment for localized cancer or lymph node metastasis, and as a palliative treatment in patients with widespread disease. Overall, nearly 50–60% of patients with cancer receive radiotherapy [8]. The role of radiotherapy in pancreatic cancer is controversial. Multiple clinical trials have been designed to access the role of radiology in pancreatic carcinoma over the last 30 years and mixed results were acquired. According to the LAP-07 trial, no benefit was found to the addition of radiotherapy to gemcitabine for locally advanced pancreatic cancer [9]. The American society of radiation oncology's (ASTRO) guidelines recommended the clinical practice of radiotherapy for high-risk pancreatic cancer patients. It is recommended to conditionally undergo fractional radiotherapy or stereotactic body radiation therapy (SBRT) after chemotherapy in surgically resectable patients. The conditional provision of conventional fractional radiation is recommended in positive lymph nodes and margins were found during surgical resection. Neoadjuvant chemotherapy combined with radiotherapy is conditionally recommended after systemic chemotherapy for patients with resectable boundaries. It is recommended to conditionally concurrent chemo or radiotherapy or SBRT as salvage radiotherapy after systemic chemotherapy in locally advanced patients who are not suitable for surgery. New radiotherapy technology, such as intensity modulated radiation therapy (IMRT), SBRT, with advances in motion management, target delineation, treatment planning, and image guidance, allows for reducing treatment-related toxicities, improving control of micro-metastatic disease and dose escalation, as well as possible synergy between radiation and other therapy. Therefore, there is great potential for radiation to improve future outcomes in pancreatic cancer [10].

2.4 Immunotherapy

Immunotherapy is a treatment that eliminates tumor cells by reactivating and enhancing the anti-tumor immune response of tumor patients. Much excitement has been generated immunotherapy in tumors that are refractory to traditional treatment, as well as resistance to traditional agents. Moreover, cancer immunotherapy has gone all the way from a promising preclinical application to a clinical reality. A variety of tumor associated antigens are high expression in pancreatic cancer, such as mucin1 (MUC-1), carcinoembryoni-cantigen (CEA), prostate stem cell antigen (PSCA), vascular endothelial growth factor (VEGF), mesoth-elin (MSLN) and K-ras mutation. Unfortunately, the use of immunotherapy alone has encountered disappointing results in clinical trials in pancreas cancer, with response rates only [10]. Immunotherapy includes the following methods: **(1) Active immunotherapy.** Active immunotherapy refers to immunizing tumor-associated antigens to stimulate tumor-specific immune response of the body to eliminate tumors. Tumor associated antigens (TAAs) have been widely explored as cancer vaccines for treatment of pancreatic cancer in both mouse models and clinical trial [11]. Due to a variety of the tumor associated antigens expressing on the pancreatic cancer cells, several vaccines can be explored for the pancreatic cancer active immunotherapy, such as GVAX vaccine. K-ras gene has a high mutation rate in pancreatic cancer and K-ras vaccine has become an important target for immunotherapy of pancreatic cancer. Studies have found that the cationic nano-encapsulated K-ras peptide vaccine has a significant therapeutic effect on pancreatic cancer xenograft mice, and can significantly prolong the survival of mice [12]. In a I phase of clinical trial, following inoculated with MUC-1 peptide-loaded DC vaccine in 7 pancreatic cancer patients, the number of mature DC cells in 2 of them increased significantly and peripheral blood lymphocytes were activated and produced large amounts of IL-12p40 and IFN-γ [13]. **(2) Passive immunotherapy.** Passive immunotherapy refers to substances with immune effects are modified in vitro and then injected into human body to enhance anti-tumor immune response and eliminate tumors. At present, passive immunotherapeutic strategies used for pancreatic cancer including: 1) Antibody-mediated passive immunotherapy. Antibody-mediated passive immunotherapy involves targeting tumors using monoclonal antibodies, antibody-drug conjugates, antibody fragments, or radio-immunotherapy conjugates to inhibit oncogenic signaling, immune suppression, or immune checkpoints [11]. Combination anti-CD40 antibody with gemcitabine showed an effective tumor inhibition. 2) Passive T cell mediated immunotherapy. Passive T cell mediated immunotherapy includes adoptive T-cell transfer and chimeric antigen receptors (CAR) T-cells therapy. **(3) Immune checkpoint blocking therapy.** Immune checkpoint blocking therapy is an immunotherapy method that can reverse the immunosuppressive signal by blocking the immunoregulatory molecules and enhance the anti-tumor immune response. Pancreatic cancer tumor cells overexpress immunosuppressive ligands, such as B7-1, B7-2 and PD-L1, which bind to surface inhibitory receptors CTL-4 and PD-1 of T cells to suppress effector T cell activity and evade immune surveillance. In 2011, the FDA approved Ipilimumab, the first humanized monoclonal antibody targeting CTL-4, for the treatment of patients with advanced melanoma. Its effect on pancreatic cancer has entered the clinical trial stage. Studies have shown that Ipilimumab can promote the proliferation of T cells and the secretion of Th1 cytokines, and enhance the killing effect of CD8+ T cells on Colo356/FG pancreatic cancer cells [14]. Two PD-1 blocking antibodies pembrolizumab and nivolumab are FDA approved for use in the treatment of metastatic non-small cell lung cancer, melanoma, renal cell cancer, and head and neck cancer [15]. In mouse model of pancreatic cancer, anti-PD-1 or PD-L1 blocking treatment promoted the generation of CD8+ T cells to tumor invasion and anti-tumor immune response. In a number of clinical trials, no objective tumor remission was observed in pancreatic cancer patients treated with anti-PD-1 or anti-PD-L1 blocking alone, suggesting that PD-1 or PD-L1 blocking alone does not have a good therapeutic effect on pancreatic cancer. **(4) CAR-T therapy.** Chimeric antigen receptor (CAR) is composed of the single chain variable fragment (ScFv) of monoclonal antibody, the hinge region and the transmembrane region of TCR receptor, and the intracellular signal transduction region in series. They form the chimeric antigen receptor by viral infection or electrical transformation on the surface of T cells. CAR-T can recognize antigens on the surface of tumor cells directly without being restricted by HLA molecules. Therefore, CAR-T has a broader application prospect in tumor immunotherapy. Target specific CAR-T cells were designed to target the highly expressed tumor-associated antigens of pancreatic cancer, making the treatment more specific. Tn-MUC-1 CAR-T: Posey et al. designed CAR-T cells targeting the Tn/STn glycopeptide phenotype on MUC-1 [16]. When CEA + C15A3 pancreatic cancer cells were transfected to mice, the cancer cells were quickly cleared and serum levels of IL-1β and IL-5 were significantly increased [17]. PSCA CAR-T: PSCA is also a tumor-associated antigen highly expressed in pancreatic cancer, and CAR-T targeting PSCA has a significant anti-tumor effect on xenograft mice of human pancreatic cancer after treatment, in which 40% of the tumors in mice have completely subsided [18]. MSLN CAR-T: Hingorani et al. designed CD8+ CAR-T cells targeting MSLN, and found that MSLN CAR-T cells could specifically kill KPC tumor cells and produce a large amount of IFN-γ in vitro. The metastasis rate dropped from 64% to 46%, and overall survival increased from 54 days to 96 days [19].

Due to unique tumor microenvironment of pancreatic cancer, both traditional treatment and single immunotherapy is not ideal. Although tumor vaccine can induce the activation of effector T cells, the activation degree is very limited and only a few effector T cells and NK cells exist in the tumor microenvironment and peripheral blood of pancreatic cancer patients. Although immune checkpoint blocking therapy can block the inhibitory effect of effector T cells, there are still many soluble immunosuppressants inhibiting effector T cells in the tumor microenvironment of pancreatic cancer. For CAR-T treatment, in addition to being influenced by immunosuppressive factors in the tumor microenvironment, the fibrous stroma layer around pancreatic cancer cells can prevent the infiltration of CAR-T into the tumor and further its efficacy. Therefore, a deep understanding the characteristics of the immune microenvironment of pancreatic cancer and its impact on immunotherapy and/or other traditional treatment will greatly improve the treatment effect. The combination of immune checkpoint blocking therapy with radiotherapy, chemotherapy and tumor vaccines can enhance the function of tumor-specific T cells and promote lymphocyte infiltration into the tumor site. Anti-CD40 agonist can reverse the resistance of pancreatic cancer mice to PD-1 and CTLA-4 blocking antibodies, and improve the therapeutic effect of blocking antibodies. Pembrolizumab (PD-1 blocking antibody) and nivolumab (CTLA-4 blocking antibody) combined with radiotherapy can significantly prolong the survival of mice with pancreatic adenocarcinoma [20]. In order to design a reasonable immunotherapy strategy according to the characteristics of pancreatic cancer microenvironment and improve the effect of pancreatic cancer immunotherapy, we should start from the following aspects: (1) destroy the fibrous matrix layer of pancreatic cancer and increase the infiltration of effector T cells into the tumor; (2) remove excessive immunosuppressive cells such as Tregs and MDSCs, and reverse the immunosuppressive microenvironment; (3) recruit more T cells to the tumor site to enhance the anti-tumor immune response of effector T cells; (4) enhance the targeting and killing of effector T cells.

3. Treatment resistance of pancreatic cancer

Radiotherapy and chemotherapy plays a central part in curing pancreatic cancer. The major cause of treatment failure with pancreatic cancer treatment strategies mainly focus on the cancer cell itself and their localized tumor microenvironment (TME). Some of the tumor cells are already resistant to the "achievable" of anticancer treatment, termed intrinsic resistance. Other tumor cells are initially sensitive but become resistant during the course of treatment, termed acquired resistance. Regardless of the intrinsic or acquired resistance mechanisms, cancer stem cells are thought to be the major cause of tumor treatment resistance. TME refers to the internal environment in which tumor cells interact with their surrounding tissue components to form a complex and conducive to the biological behavior of tumor cells.

3.1 Tumor microenvironment

Tumor microenvironment is generally composed of three parts: (1) matrix components: extracellular matrix (ECM) and stromal cells; (2) cell components: including endothelial cells and immune cells; (3) soluble factors: including cytokines and immunoregulatory molecules [21]. The components of the tumor microenvironment are conducive to tumor proliferation, invasion, adhesion, angiogenesis and anti-radiation chemotherapy, and promote the generation of malignant tumors. Pancreatic tumor microenvironment has its own characteristics: (1) a rich of matrix components, such as pancreatic stellate cells (PSC), cancer associated fibroblasts (CAF), typeI collagen, hyaluronic acid and other extracellular matrix; (2) immune cells; (3) a large number of soluble immunosuppressive factors [22].

Pancreatic cancer cells secrete platelet-derived growth factor (PDGF), transforming growth factor beta (TGF-β), AngiotensinII and other cytokines [23]. These cytokines can activate PSCs depending on several signaling pathways, such as extracellular signal-regulated kinase (ERK), c-jun nh2-terminal kinase (JNK), p38 mitogen-activated protein kinase (P38MAPK), Janus kinase-signal transducers and activators of transcription (JAK–STAT), and phosphatidylinositol 3 kinase (PI3K) [24, 25]. The activated PSCs secrete a variety of growth factors in paracrine manner, and further promote the growth and proliferation, inhibit apoptosis and enhance their invasion ability of pancreatic cancer cells, leading to the treatment resistance [26]. CAFs are the critical part of pancreatic cancer microenvironment and function in secreting extracellular matrix proteins and participating in the formation of tumor blood vessels. CAFs also secrete interferon-gamma (IFN-γ) and tumor necrosis factor-alpha (TNF-α), which further inhibits the function and infiltration of effector T cells and induces the immunotherapy failure [27]. A large amount of extracellular matrix, including collagen, fibronectin I, III, XI and hyaluronic acid exist around the pancreatic cancer cells. Extracellular matrix creates a favorable tumor microenvironment for the growth of pancreatic cancer cells [28]. Moreover, accumulated extracellular matrix leads to the collapse and occlusion of intratumoral blood vessels, making anti-tumor drugs and immune cells fail to reach the tumor, which is useful for the chemotherapy resistance and immune escape [29].

Immune cells are rich in the TME. In pancreatic cancer, the immunity is in a state of imbalance between immune cell number and function. The number of CD4 + T cells, CD8 + T cells, NK cells and DC cells is decreased and present in an inactive or immature phenotype and state. However, CD4+ regulatory T cells (Tregs), myeloid-derived suppressor cells (MDSC), and tumor associated macrophages (TAMs) with immunosuppressive effect are active and abundant [30]. The "incapacity" state of effector cells, abundance of immunosuppressive cells and their released soluble immunosuppressive factors form the immunosuppressive microenvironment of pancreatic cancer [31].

Exist of soluble immunosuppressive factors in the microenvironment of pancreatic cancer is the important mechanism for tumor cells evading immune surveillance. (1) Transforming growth factor-β (TGF-β): TGF-β is a well-studied cytokine that is secreted by various immune cells (Tregs, MDSCs and TAMs) and tumor cells [32]. TGF-β has a dual action in cancer, as a tumor suppressor and a tumor promoter. As a tumor promoter factor, TGF-β can affect both the adaptive and innate immune systems and contributes to the evasion of immune surveillance [32]. TGF-β directly inhibits CD8 + T cell cytotoxicity [33], stimulates the generation of Tregs and contributes to exclusion of T cells from the tumor core [34]. TGF-β also inhibits NK cell proliferation and cytotoxic functions and affects myeloid cells (tumor-infiltrating macrophages and neutrophils) immunosuppressive activity [35]. In addition, TGF-β also promotes pancreatic cancer progression and metastasis depending on promoting the growth of fibroblasts and the formation of tumor extracellular matrix, and inducing tumor cells to secrete VEGF and matrix metalloproteinase 2 (MMP2) [36]. (2) IL-10: IL-10 is mainly produced by Tregs and TAM and inhibits antigen presenting cell (APC) and effector T function [36]. (3) Indoleamine-2, 3-dioxygenase (IDO): IDO is mainly produced by MDSCs and pancreatic cancer cells. Its role is to catalyze the decomposition of tryptophan necessary for the activation of effector T cells into Kynurenine, thus inhibiting the activation of effector T cells [37]. Moreover, IL-10, IL-13 and IL-23 secreted by activated fibroblasts promote the transformation of CD4 + T cells into Th2 or Th17 helper T cells, which is help to the tumor immune promoter microenvironment [38]. CCL5, CCL22 and CCL17 recruit monocytes and Tregs cells to accumulate in the tumor site, which is useful for the tumor immunosuppressive microenvironment [39].

One of the most prominent features of pancreatic cancer is featured with the asymmetry distribution of nutrients, insufficient oxygenation (hypoxia), acidic pH (acidosis), and elevated levels of reactive oxygen species (ROS). Hypoxia is one of the hallmarks of pancreatic cancer and the major drivers of tumor radio and chemo-resistance. Hypoxia induces radio- or chemo-resistance through a variety of mechanisms. Firstly, hypoxia protects cancer cells from DNA damages [40, 41]. Secondly, hypoxia drives treatment resistance by accumulating and stabilizing hypoxia-inducible factor-1α (HIF-1α) [40, 42]. HIF-1a induces excessive secretion of proangiogenic signals, such as vascular endothelial growth factor (VEGF), and results in rapid but abnormal tumor vessel formation, which reduce the chemotherapy drug accumulation in the tumor bed. HIF-1α activation also increases the expression of key enzymes that drive the accumulation of lactate and pyruvate as well as the antioxidants glutathione and NADPH. NADPH scavenge reactive oxygen species (ROS) generated by radiation exposure to limit DNA damage [41]. Lactate up-regulates the HIF-1α pathway creating a futile cycle of radio- and immune resistance [42, 43]. In addition, radiation-induced vascular damage can enhance tumor hypoxia and trigger an immune response by increasing the production of cytokines/chemokines, thereby inducing the replenishment of immune cells. Subsequent tumor revascularisation occurs via HIF-1α dependent and independent recruitment of bone marrow-derived cells [44, 45].

3.2 Cancer stem cells (CSCs)

CSCs are a very small subset of relatively quiescent cells in the tumor that are endowed with the ability to self-renew and differentiate into non-stem daughter cells that make the bulk of tumor. Epigenetics has been implicated in many aspects of CSC biology and its role has been extensively studied [46]. Molecular determinants involved in various types of epigenetic modification, including DNA methylation, histone modification. Recent work has shown that miR-205 in combination with GEM was more efficient in reducing the proliferation of CSCs and resensitized GEM resistant pancreatic cancer cells to GEM [47].

Many signaling pathways are frequently deregulated in CSCs including Myc, Notch, Hedgehog (Hh), Wnt, FGF/FGFR, EGF/EGFR, NF-κB, MAPK, PTEN/PI3K, HER2, JAK/STAT and so on [48, 49]. Furthermore, altered cell cycle regulation can play a role in CSC quiescence, proliferation and apoptosis [50]. Cell cycle regulators are frequently lost (p53, Rb, p16/CDKN2A, CDKN1B) or amplified (CCND1, CDK4,CCNE1) in pancreatic CSCs [51]. Altered cell cycle program in pancreatic CSCs help them resist therapy-induced apoptosis [50].

Aside from intrinsic factors, extrinsic factors also contribute to CSC treatment resistance biology. Like normal SCs, CSCs reside in and rely on specialized tumor microenvironments, called niche, to maintain a balance between self-renewal and differentiation and therapy resistance. The CSC niche in pancreatic cancer is composed of a variety of stoma cells including inflammatory cells, immune cells, vascular endothelial cells, fibroblasts, smooth muscle cells, mesenchymal cells, adipocytes, nerve fibers and neural cells, together with extracellular matrix (ECM) [52]. These various components collaboratively interact with each other via networks of cytokines, chemokines and growth factors to create a hypoxia inflammatory, and immunosuppressive environment that facilitates pancreatic cancer treatment resistance [52]. The special pancreatic CSC niches include the hypoxia niche and the perivascular niche. In pancreatic cancer, hypoxia has been shown to promote the CSC expansion [53]. Oxygen plays a crucial role in generating ROS that mediate the anticancer effects of radiotherapy and chemotherapy. The low oxygen tensions in the hypoxia area of the tumor contain low levels of ROS, reducing the risk for the cells being killed [54]. In addition to physically protecting of the niches, other components of tumor microenvironment including extracellular matrix (ECM), cancer associated fibroblasts, immune cells and inflammatory cells also play a role in protecting pancreatic CSCs from both chemotherapy and other therapies [55]. They provide CSCs with resistant signaling stimuli through surface receptors to activate other lines of defense for CSCs. Stromal cells secrete high levels of HGF which makes co-cultured human pancreatic cancer cells acquire resistance to various anticancer drugs particularly RAF inhibitors [56]. Other growth factors or cytokines including interleukin 6 (IL-6), fibroblast growth factor (FGF) and neuregulin 1 are reported to help form the so-called 'chemo-resistant niche' of CSCs by activating various survival signaling pathways [57, 58].

In addition to the niches, CSC could activate the second line of defense under treatment stress, i.e., the drug efflux mechanisms that pump the drug out of the cell are another special defense for pancreatic CSC treatment. The transmembrane proteins of the ABCT family are the main players of drug efflux and highly expressed on pancreatic CSCs [59], including multidrug resistance-associated protein 1 (MRP1 or ABCC1) and breast cancer resistance protein (BCRP or ABCG2] [59].

In case of the drug efflux has failed and the drug has invaded the cytoplasm of CSCs, high levels of drug inactivating enzymes or low expression of the drug activating enzymes would make the cells resistant to the drugs. Thymidine phosphorylase converts capecitabine into 5-fluorouracil (5-FU) [60].

Unless unrepairable DNA damage occurs, DNA repair is another main reason for radio- or chemo-resistance of pancreatic CSCs [61, 62]. It has been shown that DNA damage checkpoint and repair proteins such as the ATM, Chk1/2,p53, BRCAs and XRCC5 are aberrantly overexpressed or over-activated in CSCs but not in non-CSCs [63], and is further activated by DNA-damaging therapy such as radiation rendering delayed cell division and prolonged DNA repair time leading to resistance [64, 65]. Similar to normal stem cells, CSCs rely on specific signaling pathways for maintaining essential proliferation, survival and the balance between self-renewal and differentiation. In response to therapies, CSCs either over-activate pro-survival and anti-apoptotic signaling or down-regulate proapoptotic signaling as another mechanism of resistance to therapies [66]. For example, inhibition of NF-κB hinders the stemness of CSCs in pancreatic cancer.

Lastly, regeneration of CSCs by EMT is a likely mechanism for radio- or chemo-resistance of cancer and relapse. EMT program has been linked to the acquisition of aggressive traits and treatment resistance in CSCs [67]. A set of pleiotropic EMT transcription factors (eg. Snail1/2, Zeb1/2, Twist) together with EMT inducers (eg. TGF-β) have been proven to contribute to CSCs treatment resistance [68]. Indeed, rapid repopulation of CSCs is believed to occur in human tumors during radiotherapy [69], and redistribution of CSCs to the quiescent phase of the cell cycle makes the cells more resistant to radiotherapy.

4. Diagnosis of pancreatic cancer

Traditional methods of diagnosing early pancreatic cancer include serum markers, imaging methods and endoscopic ultrasonography. Emerging nanotechnology and advanced materials are becoming novel strategies for pancreatic cancer diagnosis. The application of multiple diagnostic methods can help to detect pancreatic cancer in the early stage, which is help to improve the survival rate.

4.1 Serological mark

During the development of pancreatic cancer, it can actively secrete certain substances, which have been preliminarily proved to be useful for the diagnosis and prognosis evaluation of pancreatic cancer. Carbohydrate antigen 19-9(CA19-9) is the most commonly used serological marker in diagnosis of pancreatic cancer [70].

The sensitivity and specificity of CA19-9 in the diagnosis of pancreatic cancer are not high, which limits its clinical application. Combination CA19-9 with CA125 significantly improve the sensitivity of pancreatic cancer detection and contribute to its early diagnosis [71]. Dj-1, a protein secreted by pancreatic adenocarcinoma cells, was found to be positive in 68.5% of pancreatic cancer samples and significantly increased in the blood sample of pancreatic cancer patients [72]. Soluble complement iC3b was found to be able to detect tumor recurrence at the early stage and more sensitivity than imaging [73]. Recent studies have also suggested that tumor-associated antigen MUC-1 specific antibody, TAB004, may be useful in the diagnosis of pancreatic cancer [74]. In addition, combination CA19-9 with both REG4 and tumor necrosis factor-a family member, APRIL, significantly improve sensitivity to the diagnosis of pancreatic cancer [74, 75]. A recent study has shown that a serum protein biomarker panel consisting of CA125, CA19-9, and laminin γC (LAMC2) significantly improve performance in detecting pancreatic cancer than single serum marker [76].

In addition to traditional serum tumor markers, some novel circulating tumor markers has made great process. MicroRNAs are a group of small non-coding RNA, consisting of 19 to 25 nucleotides, which are involved in the growth, proliferation and differentiation of pancreatic cancer. Multiple studies have confirmed that abnormally expressed serum microRNAs, such as miR-21, miR-196a and miR-155, have certain significance in the diagnosis of pancreatic cancer. Moreover, the diagnostic value of microRNAs is higher than that of traditional serum tumor markers [77]. Exosome is a kind of extracellular vesicles (EV), with a size of 50 ~ 150 nm. Exosome can be secreted under physiological or pathological state. Exosome contains DNA, microRNA, protein or other signaling molecules, and plays the role of exchanging information between cells. Since tumor cells can secrete exosomes 10 times more than normal cells, analysis of abnormal serum exosomes and their encapsulated molecules often has widely been application in the diagnosis for tumors [78]. With the ability to enter the peripheral circulatory system, circulatory tumor cells (CTC) vary in individual and express both epithelial and mesenchymal markers [79]. It has been reported that such cells can be detected in the peripheral blood of 40% ~ 100% of pancreatic cancer patients, which may be used for the early diagnosis of pancreatic cancer [80].

4.2 Imaging diagnosis

Multi-Detector Computed Tomography (MDCT) is now the most routinely performed for the diagnosis of suspicious pancreatic lesions, assessment of resectability and vascular invasion, and detecting metastatic lesions [81]. The appearances of pancreatic cancer in non-contrast CT scan include solid mass (84.2%), diffuse enlargement (13.3%) with a vague or uneven glandular appearance, usually of slightly lower or equal density. A pancreas-specific protocol with dual-phase or multi-phase dynamic contrast is usually used, including early arterial phase images, pancreatic phase images and portal venous phase images. Early arterial phase images are sensitivity in evaluating the tumor and peri-pancreatic arteries. Pancreatic phase images are sensitivity in evaluating pancreatic lesions, and portal venous phase images are sensitivity in evaluating the involvement of the portal vein, the superior mesenteric vein and other veins. Enhanced CT scan showed enhancement in the early stage, with a peak earlier than the liver, relative lack of blood, about 93% showed uneven low density, distal pancreatic atrophy and dilatation of the pancreatic duct [81].

In addition to showing the anatomical features of pancreatic tumors, MRI can also supply information about the metastatic lesions in lymph nodes and liver.

The weighted expression of T1WI was low or slightly low signal, while T2WI was slightly high or mixed signal for the tumor mass. The enhancement scan showed significant enhancement of the normal pancreas and only slight enhancement of the tumor. Diffusion-weighted imaging (DWI) is an MRI technique based on the Brownian motion of water molecules in tissue [82], which is greatly useful in differentiating mass-forming focal pancreatitis from pancreatic cancer [83, 84].

PET-CT can show the metabolic activity of the tumor, and has obvious advantages in the detection of pancreatic metastasis and the evaluation of systemic tumor load. Combination of PET-CT with endoscopic ultrasonography is useful for suspected pancreatic cancer diagnosis because of the high sensitivity of PET-CT and the high specificity of endoscopic ultrasonography (EUS) [85].

EUS is considered the most sensitive method for detecting early neoplastic in the pancreas, which is superior to MDCT [86]. A meta-analysis of 20 studies showed that the performance of EUS in PDAC diagnosis depended on the T stage. The sensitivity and specificity was 72% and 90% for T1–2 stage cancers and 90% and 72% for T3–4 stage cancer in EUS [87]. EUS can detect pancreas lesions as small as 2–3 mm [88]. In particular, EUS guided fine needle biopsy has become the most accurate method for the localization and qualitative diagnosis of pancreatic cancer.

4.3 Molecular imaging diagnosis

In 1999, Weissleder of Harvard University first proposed the concept of molecular imaging [89]. Molecular imaging is a biological process that can be observed, qualitatively and quantitatively analyzed in humans and other living organisms at the molecular or cellular level. It generally includes two-dimensional or three-dimensional images and quantitative maps of signals changing over time. The rise of molecular imaging has broken the limitation of traditional imaging in mainly reflecting the changes of anatomical structure, made modern medical imaging go deep into the microscopic level of living organisms, realized the extension of structural image to functional image, and provided an effective way for accurate medical disease diagnosis. Molecular imaging relies on advanced imaging equipment, highly sensitive and specific molecular imaging probes [89].

Several groups have investigated novel imaging agents that are coupled to 18F applied to PET own to its false positives (eg, benign causes of inflammation like pancreatitis) and false negatives (eg, non–18F fluorodeoxyglucose avid tumors). Other strategies to detect pancreatic cancer with molecular imaging agents include targeting proteins that are overexpressed by the cancer (eg, mesothelin), signaling pathways (eg, epidermal growth factor receptor), tumor stroma (eg, hedgehog signaling, vascular endothelial growth factor), and other targets that are associated with the disease (eg, plectin-1, MUC-1] [90]. Another molecular imaging method that is of interest for early detection is hyperpolarized MRI, which can identify metabolic aberrations in the pancreas that indicate precancerous lesions [91].

Researchers used PEG as shell, limiting Mn^{2+} calcium phosphate acid as nuclear build a lack of oxygen can be used in the tumor area imaging of molecular probes, after the probe enters the tumor, tumor area lower pH can cause lack of oxygen. The dissolution of calcium phosphate thus releases its limitations of Mn^{2+}, causing local T1 relaxation rate increase significantly, thus successfully mapping the hypoxia zone in the tumor to improve clinical tumor treatment effect [92]. In addition, the design of introducing the disulfide bond into the probe and being interrupted by increased glutathione (GSH) in vivo successfully realized the molecular level imaging (fluorescence, 19f-MRS, MRI, etc.) reflecting the redox state of the lesion area [93]. By introducing amino acid sequences that can be recognized and cut off by caspase-3, the probe can realize the aggregation of small molecule monomers under the action of activated caspase-3, causing significant amplification of the imaging signal, and thus reflecting the occurrence of early apoptotic events in pancreatic carcinoma [94].

5. Conclusion

As one of the highest mortality cancer, pancreatic cancer is still a disaster disease. Novel diagnosis and therapy avenues should be developed to improve the survival rate of this disease.

Acknowledgements

The authors acknowledge financial support from the Natural Science Foundation of Jiangsu Province (Grant no. BK20191223), Key Programme of Jiangsu Commission of Health (Grant no. K2019024), Six talent peals project of Jiangsu Province (Grant No.WSW-039), Six for one project of Jiangsu Province (Grant No. LGY2018093), Young medical talents of Jiangsu (Grant No. QNRC2016833), Project of China International Medical Foundation SKY Medical Imaging (Z-2014-2107-1912-1918).

Author details

Xiaojie Cai[1,2], Jie Gao[1], Yanfang Liu[3], Ming Wang[1], Qiulian Ma[1], Aihua Gong[3], Dongqing Wang[1] and Haitao Zhu[1*]

1 Department of Medical Imaging, The Affiliated Hospital of Jiangsu University, Zhenjiang, China

2 Department of Radiology, Changshu Hospital Affiliated to Soochow University, First People's Hospital of Changshu City, China

3 School of Medicine, Jiangsu University, Zhenjiang, China

*Address all correspondence to: zhht25@163.com

References

[1] Rahib L, Smith BD, Aizenberg R, Rosenzweig AB, Fleshman JM, Matrisian LM. Projecting cancer incidence and deaths to 2030: the unexpected burden of thyroid, liver, and pancreas cancers in the United States. Cancer research. 2014;**74**(11):2913-2921

[2] American Cancer Society. Cancer Facts and Figures 2018.

[3] National Comprehensive Cancer Network (NCCN) guidelines 2018.

[4] Terumi Kamisawa, Laura D. Wood, Takao Itoi, Kyoichi Takaori. Pancreatic cancer. The Lancet. 2016;**388**(10039):73-85.

[5] Ryan DP, Hong TS, Bardeesy N. Pancreatic adenocarcinoma. N Engl J Med. 2014;**371**(11):1039-1049.

[6] Conroy T, Desseigne F, Ychou M, Bouché O, Guimbaud R, Bécouarn Y, Adenis A, Raoul JL, Gourgou-Bourgade S, de la Fouchardière C, BennounaJ, BachetJB, Khemissa-AkouzF, Péré-Vergé D, Delbaldo C, Assenat E, Chauffert B, Michel P, Montoto-Grillot C, Ducreux M. FOLFIRINOX versus gemcitabine for metastatic pancreatic cancer. N Engl J Med. 2011;**364**(19):1817-1825.

[7] Von Hoff DD, Ramanathan RK, Borad MJ, Laheru DA, Smith LS, Wood TE, Korn RL, Desai N, Trieu V, Iglesias JL, Zhang H, Soon-Shiong P, Shi T, Rajeshkumar NV, Maitra A, Hidalgo M. Gemcitabine plus nab-paclitaxel is an active regimen in patients with advanced pancreatic cancer: a phase I/II trial. Journal of clinical oncology : official journal of the American Society of Clinical Oncology. 2011;**29**(34):4548-4554.

[8] G. Delaney, S. Jacob, C. Featherstone, M. Barton. The role of radiotherapy in cancer treatment: estimating optimal utilization from a review of evidence-based clinical guidelines. Cancer. 2005;**104**(6):1129-1137.

[9] Hammel P, Huguet F, van Laethem JL, Goldstein D, Glimelius B, Artru P, Borbath I, Bouché O, Shannon J, André T, Mineur L, Chibaudel B, Bonnetain F, Louvet C. Effect of Chemoradiotherapy vs Chemotherapy on Survival in Patients With Locally Advanced Pancreatic Cancer Controlled After 4 Months of Gemcitabine With or Without Erlotinib: The LAP07 Randomized Clinical Trial. JAMA. 2016;**315**(17):1844-1853.

[10] Palta M, Godfrey D, Goodman KA, Hoffe S, Dawson LA, Dessert D, Hall WA, Herman JM, Khorana AA, Merchant N, Parekh A, Patton C, Pepek JM, Salama JK, Tuli R, Koong AC. Radiation Therapy for Pancreatic Cancer: Executive Summary of an ASTRO Clinical Practice Guideline. Pract Radiat Oncol. 2019;**9**(5):322-332.

[11] Banerjee K, Kumar S, Ross KA, Gautam S, Poelaert B, Nasser MW, Aithal A, Bhatia R, Wannemuehler MJ, Narasimhan B, Solheim JC, Batra SK, Jain M. Emerging trends in the immunotherapy of pancreatic cancer. Cancer letters. 2018;**417**:35-46.

[12] Tan G, Wang Z, Zhang X, Cai Z, Zhang J. Induction of CTLs by DCs pulsed with K-ras mutant peptide on the surface of nanoparticles in the treatment of pancreatic cancer. Oncology reports. 2011;**26**(1):215-221.

[13] Rong Y, Qin X, Jin D, Lou W, Wu L, Wang D, Wu W, Ni X, Mao Z, Kuang T, Zang YQ, Qin X. A phase I pilot trial of MUC1-peptide-pulsed dendritic cells in the treatment of advanced pancreatic cancer. Clinical and experimental medicine. 2012;**12**(3):173-180.

[14] Yano H, Thakur A, Tomaszewski EN, Choi M,

Deol A, Lum LG. Ipilimumab augments antitumor activity of bispecific antibody-armed T cells. Journal of translational medicine. 2014;**12**(undefined):191.

[15] Byrne KT, Vonderheide RH, Jaffee EM, Armstrong TD. Special Conference on Tumor Immunology and Immunotherapy: A New Chapter. Cancer immunology research. 2015;**3**(6):590-597.

[16] Avery D Posey, Henrik Clausen, Carl H June. Distinguishing Truncated and Normal MUC1 Glycoform Targeting from Tn-MUC1-Specific CAR T Cells: Specificity Is the Key to Safety. Immunity. 2016;**45**(5):947-948.

[17] Chmielewski M, Hahn O, Rappl G, Nowak M, Schmidt-Wolf IH, Hombach AA, Abken H. T cells that target carcinoembryonic antigen eradicate orthotopic pancreatic carcinomas without inducing autoimmune colitis in mice. Gastroenterology. 2012;**143**(4):1095-1107.e1092.

[18] Abate-Daga D, Lagisetty KH, Tran E, Zheng Z, Gattinoni L, Yu Z, Burns WR, Miermont AM, Teper Y, Rudloff U, Restifo NP, Feldman SA, Rosenberg SA, Morgan RA. A novel chimeric antigen receptor against prostate stem cell antigen mediates tumor destruction in a humanized mouse model of pancreatic cancer. Human gene therapy. 2014;**25**(12):1003-1012.

[19] Stromnes IM, Schmitt TM, Hulbert A, Brockenbrough JS, Nguyen H, Cuevas C, Dotson AM, Tan X, Hotes JL, Greenberg PD, Hingorani SR. T Cells Engineered against a Native Antigen Can Surmount Immunologic and Physical Barriers to Treat Pancreatic Ductal Adenocarcinoma. Cancer cell. 2015;**28**(5):638-652.

[20] Winograd R, Byrne KT, Evans RA, Odorizzi PM, Meyer AR, Bajor DL, Clendenin C, Stanger BZ, Furth EE, Wherry EJ, Vonderheide RH. Induction of T-cell Immunity Overcomes Complete Resistance to PD-1 and CTLA-4 Blockade and Improves Survival in Pancreatic Carcinoma. Cancer immunology research. 2015;**3**(4):399-411.

[21] Mittal K, Ebos J, Rini B. Angiogenesis and the tumor microenvironment: vascular endothelial growth factor and beyond. Seminars in oncology. 2014;**41**(2):235-251.

[22] Neesse A, Frese KK, Bapiro TE, Nakagawa T, Sternlicht MD, Seeley TW, Pilarsky C, Jodrell DI, Spong SM, Tuveson DA. CTGF antagonism with mAb FG-3019 enhances chemotherapy response without increasing drug delivery in murine ductal pancreas cancer. Proceedings of the National Academy of Sciences of the United States of America. 2013;**110**(30):12325-12330.

[23] Mews P, Phillips P, Fahmy R, Korsten M, Pirola R, Wilson J, Apte M. Pancreatic stellate cells respond to inflammatory cytokines: potential role in chronic pancreatitis. Gut. 2002;**50**(4):535-541.

[24] Jaster R, Sparmann G, Emmrich J, Liebe S. Extracellular signal regulated kinases are key mediators of mitogenic signals in rat pancreatic stellate cells. Gut. 2002;**51**(4):579-584.

[25] Masamune A, Kikuta K, Suzuki N, Satoh M, Satoh K, Shimosegawa T. A c-Jun NH2-terminal kinase inhibitor SP600125 (anthra[1,9-cd]pyrazole-6 (2H)-one) blocks activation of pancreatic stellate cells. The Journal of pharmacology and experimental therapeutics. 2004;**310**(2):520-527.

[26] Mendelsohn J, Baselga J. The EGF receptor family as targets for cancer therapy. Oncogene. 2000;**19**(56):6550-6565.

[27] Kraman M, Bambrough PJ, Arnold JN, Roberts EW, Magiera L, Jones JO, Gopinathan A, Tuveson DA, Fearon DT. Suppression of antitumor immunity by stromal cells expressing fibroblast activation protein-alpha. Science (New York, NY). 2010;**330**(6005):827-830.

[28] Haqq J, Howells LM, Garcea G, Metcalfe MS, Steward WP, Dennison AR. Pancreatic stellate cells and pancreas cancer: current perspectives and future strategies. European journal of cancer (Oxford, England : 1990). 2014;**50**(15):2570-2582.

[29] Neesse A, Michl P, Frese KK, Feig C, Cook N, Jacobetz MA, Lolkema MP, Buchholz M, Olive KP, Gress TM, Tuveson DA. Stromal biology and therapy in pancreatic cancer. Gut. 2011;**60**(6):861-868.

[30] Murakami T, Hiroshima Y, Matsuyama R, Homma Y, Hoffman RM, Endo I. Role of the tumor microenvironment in pancreatic cancer. Annals of gastroenterological surgery. 2019;**3**(2):130-137.

[31] Looi CK, Chung FF, Leong CO, Wong SF, Rosli R, Mai CW. Therapeutic challenges and current immunomodulatory strategies in targeting the immunosuppressive pancreatic tumor microenvironment. Journal of experimental & clinical cancer research : CR. 2019;**38**(1):162.

[32] Colak S, Ten Dijke P. Targeting TGF-β Signaling in Cancer. Trends in cancer. 2017;**3**(1):56-71.

[33] Thomas DA, Massagué J. TGF-beta directly targets cytotoxic T cell functions during tumor evasion of immune surveillance. Cancer cell. 2005;**8**(5):369-380.

[34] Mariathasan S, Turley SJ, Nickles D, Castiglioni A, Yuen K, Wang Y, Kadel EE, Koeppen H, Astarita JL, Cubas R, Jhunjhunwala S, Banchereau R, Yang Y, Guan Y, Chalouni C, Ziai J, Şenbabaoğlu Y, Santoro S, Sheinson D, Hung J, Giltnane JM, Pierce AA, Mesh K, Lianoglou S, Riegler J, Carano RAD, Eriksson P, Höglund M, Somarriba L, Halligan DL, van der Heijden MS, Loriot Y, Rosenberg JE, Fong L, Mellman I, Chen DS, Green M, Derleth C, Fine GD, Hegde PS, Bourgon R, Powles T. TGFβ attenuates tumour response to PD-L1 blockade by contributing to exclusion of T cells. Nature. 2018;**554**(7693):544-548.

[35] Ghiringhelli F, Puig PE, Roux S, Parcellier A, Schmitt E, Solary E, Kroemer G, Martin F, Chauffert B, Zitvogel L. Tumor cells convert immature myeloid dendritic cells into TGF-beta-secreting cells inducing CD4+CD25+ regulatory T cell proliferation. The Journal of experimental medicine. 2005;**202**(7):919-929.

[36] Ren B, Cui M, Yang G, Wang H, Feng M, You L, Zhao Y. Tumor microenvironment participates in metastasis of pancreatic cancer. Molecular cancer. 2018;**17**(1):108.

[37] Uyttenhove C, Pilotte L, Théate I, Stroobant V, Colau D, Parmentier N, Boon T, Van den Eynde BJ. Evidence for a tumoral immune resistance mechanism based on tryptophan degradation by indoleamine 2,3-dioxygenase. Nature medicine. 2003;**9**(10):1269-1274.

[38] S Leung, X Liu, L Fang, X Chen, T Guo, J Zhang. The cytokine milieu in the interplay of pathogenic Th1/Th17 cells and regulatory T cells in autoimmune disease. Cellular & molecular immunology. 2010;**7**(3):182-189.

[39] De Monte L, Reni M, Tassi E, Clavenna D, Papa I, Recalde H, Braga M, Di Carlo V, Doglioni C, Protti MP. Intratumor T helper type 2 cell infiltrate correlates with cancer-associated fibroblast thymic stromal lymphopoietin production and reduced

survival in pancreatic cancer. The Journal of experimental medicine. 2011;**208**(3):469-478.

[40] Rockwell S, Dobrucki IT, Kim EY, Marrison ST, Vu VT. Hypoxia and radiation therapy: past history, ongoing research, and future promise. Current molecular medicine. 2009;**9**(4):442-458.

[41] Meijer TW, Kaanders JH, Span PN, Bussink J. Targeting hypoxia, HIF-1, and tumor glucose metabolism to improve radiotherapy efficacy. Clinical cancer research : an official journal of the American Association for Cancer Research. 2012;**18**(20):5585-5594.

[42] Carlson DJ, Yenice KM, Orton CG. Tumor hypoxia is an important mechanism of radioresistance in hypofractionated radiotherapy and must be considered in the treatment planning process. Medical physics. 2011;**38**(12):6347-6350.

[43] Lee DC, Sohn HA, Park ZY, Oh S, Kang YK, Lee KM, Kang M, Jang YJ, Yang SJ, Hong YK, Noh H, Kim JA, Kim DJ, Bae KH, Kim DM, Chung SJ, Yoo HS, Yu DY, Park KC, Yeom YI. A lactate-induced response to hypoxia. Cell. 2015;**161**(3):595-609.

[44] Begg AC, Stewart FA, Vens C. Strategies to improve radiotherapy with targeted drugs. Nature reviews Cancer. 2011;**11**(4):239-253.

[45] Lerman OZ, Greives MR, Singh SP, Thanik VD, Chang CC, Seiser N, Brown DJ, Knobel D, Schneider RJ, Formenti SC, Saadeh PB, Levine JP. Low-dose radiation augments vasculogenesis signaling through HIF-1-dependent and -independent SDF-1 induction. Blood. 2010;**116**(18):3669-3676.

[46] Chen T, Dent SY. Chromatin modifiers and remodellers: regulators of cellular differentiation. Nature reviews Genetics. 2014;**15**(2):93-106.

[47] Chaudhary AK, Mondal G, Kumar V, Kattel K, Mahato RI. Chemosensitization and inhibition of pancreatic cancer stem cell proliferation by overexpression of microRNA-205. Cancer letters. 2017;**402**:1-8.

[48] Okamoto OK. Cancer stem cell genomics: the quest for early markers of malignant progression. Expert review of molecular diagnostics. 2009;**9**(6):545-554.

[49] Regenbrecht CR, Lehrach H, Adjaye J. Stemming cancer: functional genomics of cancer stem cells in solid tumors. Stem cell reviews. 2008;**4**(4):319-328.

[50] Chappell J, Dalton S. Altered cell cycle regulation helps stem-like carcinoma cells resist apoptosis. BMC biology. 2010;**8**(undefined):63.

[51] Helsten T, Kato S, Schwaederle M, Tomson BN, Buys TP, Elkin SK, Carter JL, Kurzrock R. Cell-Cycle Gene Alterations in 4,864 Tumors Analyzed by Next-Generation Sequencing: Implications for Targeted Therapeutics. Molecular cancer therapeutics. 2016;**15**(7):1682-1690.

[52] Plaks V, Kong N, Werb Z. The cancer stem cell niche: how essential is the niche in regulating stemness of tumor cells? Cell stem cell. 2015;**16**(3):225-238.

[53] Hashimoto O, Shimizu K, Semba S, Chiba S, Ku Y, Yokozaki H, Hori Y. Hypoxia induces tumor aggressiveness and the expansion of CD133-positive cells in a hypoxia-inducible factor-1α-dependent manner in pancreatic cancer cells. Pathobiology : journal of immunopathology, molecular and cellular biology. 2011;**78**(4):181-192.

[54] Brown JM, Wilson WR. Exploiting tumour hypoxia in cancer treatment. Nature reviews Cancer. 2004;**4**(6):437-447.

[55] McMillin DW, Negri JM, Mitsiades CS. The role of tumour-stromal interactions in modifying drug response: challenges and opportunities. Nature reviews Drug discovery. 2013;**12**(3):217-228.

[56] Straussman R, Morikawa T, Shee K, Barzily-Rokni M, Qian ZR, Du J, Davis A, Mongare MM, Gould J, Frederick DT, Cooper ZA, Chapman PB, Solit DB, Ribas A, Lo RS, Flaherty KT, Ogino S, Wargo JA, Golub TR. Tumour micro-environment elicits innate resistance to RAF inhibitors through HGF secretion. Nature. 2012;**487**(7408):500-504.

[57] Gilbert LA, Hemann MT. DNA damage-mediated induction of a chemoresistant niche. Cell. 2010;**143**(3):355-366.

[58] Wilson TR, Fridlyand J, Yan Y, Penuel E, Burton L, Chan E, Peng J, Lin E, Wang Y, Sosman J, Ribas A, Li J, Moffat J, Sutherlin DP, Koeppen H, Merchant M, Neve R, Settleman J. Widespread potential for growth-factor-driven resistance to anticancer kinase inhibitors. Nature. 2012;**487**(7408):505-509.

[59] Gottesman MM, Fojo T, Bates SE. Multidrug resistance in cancer: role of ATP-dependent transporters. Nature reviews Cancer. 2002;**2**(1):48-58.

[60] Malet-Martino M, Martino R. Clinical studies of three oral prodrugs of 5-fluorouracil (capecitabine, UFT, S-1): a review. The oncologist. 2002;**7**(4):288-323.

[61] Bouwman P, Jonkers J. The effects of deregulated DNA damage signalling on cancer chemotherapy response and resistance. Nature reviews Cancer. 2012;**12**(9):587-598.

[62] Pajonk F, Vlashi E, McBride WH. Radiation resistance of cancer stem cells: the 4 R's of radiobiology revisited. Stem cells (Dayton, Ohio). 2010;**28**(4):639-648.

[63] Zhang M, Behbod F, Atkinson RL, Landis MD, Kittrell F, Edwards D, Medina D, Tsimelzon A, Hilsenbeck S, Green JE, Michalowska AM, Rosen JM. Identification of tumor-initiating cells in a p53-null mouse model of breast cancer. Cancer research. 2008;**68**(12):4674-4682.

[64] Squatrito M, Brennan CW, Helmy K, Huse JT, Petrini JH, Holland EC. Loss of ATM/Chk2/p53 pathway components accelerates tumor development and contributes to radiation resistance in gliomas. Cancer cell. 2010;**18**(6):619-629.

[65] Ropolo M, Daga A, Griffero F, Foresta M, Casartelli G, Zunino A, Poggi A, Cappelli E, Zona G, Spaziante R, Corte G, Frosina G. Comparative analysis of DNA repair in stem and nonstem glioma cell cultures. Molecular cancer research : MCR. 2009;**7**(3):383-392.

[66] Sun L, Mathews LA, Cabarcas SM, Zhang X, Yang A, Zhang Y, Young MR, Klarmann KD, Keller JR, Farrar WL. Epigenetic regulation of SOX9 by the NF-κB signaling pathway in pancreatic cancer stem cells. Stem cells (Dayton, Ohio). 2013;**31**(8):1454-1466.

[67] Mani SA, Guo W, Liao MJ, Eaton EN, Ayyanan A, Zhou AY, Brooks M, Reinhard F, Zhang CC, Shipitsin M, Campbell LL, Polyak K, Brisken C, Yang J, Weinberg RA. The epithelial-mesenchymal transition generates cells with properties of stem cells. Cell. 2008;**133**(4):704-715.

[68] Scheel C, Weinberg RA. Cancer stem cells and epithelial-mesenchymal transition: concepts and molecular links. Seminars in cancer biology. 2012;**22**(null):396-403.

[69] Miyabayashi T, Teo JL, Yamamoto M, McMillan M, Nguyen C, Kahn M. Wnt/beta-catenin/CBP signaling maintains long-term murine embryonic stem cell pluripotency. Proceedings of the National Academy of Sciences of the United States of America. 2007;**104**(13):5668-5673.

[70] Chakraborty S, Baine MJ, Sasson AR, Batra SK. Current status of molecular markers for early detection of sporadic pancreatic cancer. Biochimica et biophysica acta. 2011;**1815**(1):44-64.

[71] O'Brien DP, Sandanayake NS, Jenkinson C, Gentry-Maharaj A, ApostolidouS,FourkalaEO,CamuzeauxS, Blyuss O, Gunu R, Dawnay A, Zaikin A, Smith RC, Jacobs IJ, Menon U, Costello E, Pereira SP, Timms JF. Serum CA19-9 is significantly upregulated up to 2 years before diagnosis with pancreatic cancer: implications for early disease detection. Clinical cancer research : an official journal of the American Association for Cancer Research. 2015;**21**(3):622-631.

[72] He X, Zheng Z, Li J, Ben Q, Liu J, Zhang J, Ji J, Yu B, Chen X, Su L, Zhou L, Liu B, Yuan Y. DJ-1 promotes invasion and metastasis of pancreatic cancer cells by activating SRC/ERK/uPA. Carcinogenesis. 2012;**33**(3):555-562.

[73] Märten A, Büchler MW, Werft W, Wente MN, Kirschfink M, Schmidt J. Soluble iC3b as an early marker for pancreatic adenocarcinoma is superior to CA19.9 and radiology. Journal of immunotherapy (Hagerstown, Md : 1997). 2010;**33**(2):219-224.

[74] Wu ST, Williams CD, Grover PA, Moore LJ, Mukherjee P. Early detection of pancreatic cancer in mouse models using a novel antibody, TAB004. PloS one. 2018;**13**(2):e0193260.

[75] Conrad C, Fernández-Del Castillo C. Preoperative evaluation and management of the pancreatic head mass. Journal of surgical oncology. 2013;**107**(1):23-32.

[76] Chan A, Prassas I, Dimitromanolakis A, Brand RE, Serra S, Diamandis EP, Blasutig IM. Validation of biomarkers that complement CA19.9 in detecting early pancreatic cancer. Clinical cancer research : an official journal of the American Association for Cancer Research. 2014;**20**(22):5787-5795.

[77] Johansen JS, Calatayud D, Albieri V, Schultz NA, Dehlendorff C, Werner J, Jensen BV, Pfeiffer P, Bojesen SE, Giese N, Nielsen KR, Nielsen SE, Yilmaz M, Holländer NH, Andersen KK. The potential diagnostic value of serum microRNA signature in patients with pancreatic cancer. International journal of cancer. 2016;**139**(10):2312-2324.

[78] Melo SA, Luecke LB, Kahlert C, Fernandez AF, Gammon ST, Kaye J, LeBleu VS, Mittendorf EA, Weitz J, Rahbari N, Reissfelder C, Pilarsky C, Fraga MF, Piwnica-Worms D, Kalluri R. Glypican-1 identifies cancer exosomes and detects early pancreatic cancer. Nature. 2015;**523**(7559):177-182.

[79] Barriere G, Fici P, Gallerani G, Fabbri F, Zoli W, Rigaud M. Circulating tumor cells and epithelial, mesenchymal and stemness markers: characterization of cell subpopulations. Annals of translational medicine. 2014;**2**(11):109.

[80] Martini V, Timme-Bronsert S, Fichtner-Feigl S, Hoeppner J, Kulemann B. Circulating Tumor Cells in Pancreatic Cancer: Current Perspectives. Cancers. 2019;**11**(11).

[81] Zhang Y, Huang J, Chen M, Jiao LR. Preoperative vascular evaluation with computed tomography and magnetic resonance imaging for pancreatic cancer: a meta-analysis. Pancreatology: official journal of the International Association of Pancreatology (IAP) [et al]. 2012;**12**(3):227-233.

[82] Balci NC, Perman WH, Saglam S, Akisik F, Fattahi R, Bilgin M. Diffusion-weighted magnetic resonance imaging of the pancreas. Topics in magnetic resonance imaging : TMRI. 2009;**20**(1):43-47.

[83] Takeuchi M, Matsuzaki K, Kubo H, Nishitani H. High-b-value diffusion-weighted magnetic resonance imaging of pancreatic cancer and mass-forming chronic pancreatitis: preliminary results. Acta radiologica (Stockholm, Sweden : 1987). 2008;**49**(4):383-386.

[84] Fattahi R, Balci NC, Perman WH, Hsueh EC, Alkaade S, Havlioglu N, Burton FR. Pancreatic diffusion-weighted imaging (DWI): comparison between mass-forming focal pancreatitis (FP), pancreatic cancer (PC), and normal pancreas. Journal of magnetic resonance imaging : JMRI. 2009;**29**(2):350-356.

[85] Tang S, Huang G, Liu J, Liu T, Treven L, Song S, Zhang C, Pan L, Zhang T. Usefulness of 18F-FDG PET, combined FDG-PET/CT and EUS in diagnosing primary pancreatic carcinoma: a meta-analysis. European journal of radiology. 2011;**78**(1):142-150.

[86] DeWitt J, Devereaux B, Chriswell M, McGreevy K, Howard T, Imperiale TF, Ciaccia D, Lane KA, Maglinte D, Kopecky K, LeBlanc J, McHenry L, Madura J, Aisen A, Cramer H, Cummings O, Sherman S. Comparison of endoscopic ultrasonography and multidetector computed tomography for detecting and staging pancreatic cancer. Annals of internal medicine. 2004;**141**(10):753-763.

[87] Li JH, He R, Li YM, Cao G, Ma QY, Yang WB. Endoscopic ultrasonography for tumor node staging and vascular invasion in pancreatic cancer: a meta-analysis. Digestive surgery. 2014;**31**(null):297-305.

[88] Minniti S, Bruno C, Biasiutti C, Tonel D, Falzone A, Falconi M, Procacci C. Sonography versus helical CT in identification and staging of pancreatic ductal adenocarcinoma. Journal of clinical ultrasound : JCU. 2003;**31**(4):175-182.

[89] Weissleder R. Molecular imaging: exploring the next frontier. Radiology. 1999;**212**(3):609-614.

[90] England CG, Hernandez R, Eddine SB, Cai W. Molecular Imaging of Pancreatic Cancer with Antibodies. Molecular pharmaceutics. 2016;**13**(1):8-24.

[91] Serrao EM, Kettunen MI, Rodrigues TB, Dzien P, Wright AJ, Gopinathan A, Gallagher FA, Lewis DY, Frese KK, Almeida J, Howat WJ, Tuveson DA, Brindle KM. MRI with hyperpolarised [1-13C]pyruvate detects advanced pancreatic preneoplasia prior to invasive disease in a mouse model. Gut. 2016;**65**(3):465-475.

[92] Mi P, Kokuryo D, Cabral H, Wu H, Terada Y, Saga T, Aoki I, Nishiyama N, Kataoka K. A pH-activatable nanoparticle with signal-amplification capabilities for non-invasive imaging of tumour malignancy. Nature nanotechnology. 2016;**11**(8):724-730.

[93] Zheng M, Wang Y, Shi H, Hu Y, Feng L, Luo Z, Zhou M, He J, Zhou Z, Zhang Y, Ye D. Redox-Mediated Disassembly to Build Activatable

Trimodal Probe for Molecular Imaging of Biothiols. ACS nano. 2016;**10**(11):10075-10085.

[94] Yuan Y, Ding Z, Qian J, Zhang J, Xu J, Dong X, Han T, Ge S, Luo Y, Wang Y, Zhong K, Liang G. Casp3/7-Instructed Intracellular Aggregation of Fe3O4 Nanoparticles Enhances T2 MR Imaging of Tumor Apoptosis. Nano letters. 2016;**16**(4):2686-2691.

Chapter 3

KRas4BG12C/D/PDE6δ Heterodimeric Molecular Complex: A Target Molecular Multicomplex for the Identification and Evaluation of Nontoxic Pharmacological Compounds for the Treatment of Pancreatic Cancer

Paola Briseño-Díaz, Dora Emma Velez-Uriza, Pedro Cruz-Nova, Martiniano Bello Ramirez, Jose Correa-Basurto, Rosaura Hernandez-Rivas, Ma del Rocio Thompson Bonilla and Miguel Ángel Vargas Mejía

Abstract

The search for new targeted therapies to improve the quality of life of patients with pancreatic cancer has taken about 30 years. Compounds that can inhibit the K-Ras4B oncoprotein signaling pathway have been sought. Taking into account that the interaction of KRas4B with PDE6δ is essential for its transport and subsequent activation in the plasma membrane, our working group identified and evaluated in vitro and in vivo small organic molecules that could act as molecular staples to stabilize the KRas4B/PDE6δ heterodimeric complex. From this group of molecules, 38 compounds with high interaction energies on the structure of the crystallized molecular complex were selected, indicating that they efficiently stabilized the molecular complex. In vitro evaluation of compounds called D14, C22, and C19 showed significant specific effects on the cell viability of pancreatic cancer cells (and not on normal cells), thus inducing death by apoptosis and significantly inhibiting the activation of the pathways, signaling AKT and ERK. In addition to these experimental findings, we were also able to detect that compounds D14 and C22 showed significant tumor growth inhibitory activity in pancreatic cancer cell-induced subcutaneous xenograft models.

Keywords: KRas4B, PDE6, therapy

1. Introduction

About 95% of the pancreatic ductal adenocarcinoma (PDAC) originates in the exocrine pancreas, and 5% is generated in the endocrine pancreas. There are several precursors for the development of PDAC; among them, noninfiltrating lesions, called pancreatic intraepithelial neoplasia or PanIN [1], are remarkable. The follow-up of the PanIN toward an infiltrating lesion is given by the abnormal distribution inside the pancreas. These lesions can be located in the pancreatic parenchyma, which causes its infiltration. Currently, the development of a pancreatic adenocarcinoma is monitored by measuring the overexpression of EGFR, KRAS, MUC1, and MUC4 genes or the inactivation of INK4A, TP53, and BRCA2 genes, which are essential for proper cell functioning [1–4, 5–8].

The invasive ductal adenocarcinoma is the most common pancreatic neoplasm, as it occurs in 85% of the cases. Eighty percent of the patients with this type of neoplasm have an average survival of 3–6 months after the detection; that is why this adenocarcinoma has been proposed as one of the most deadly existing [1, 9–11]. The invasive micro ductal adenocarcinoma deforms the small pancreatic glands, infiltrates the stroma, and triggers a fibrous coating, where 98% of the cases present mutations in the KRas4B gene [2, 10]. One of the most important factors for the development, maintenance, and progression of this disease is the presence of mutations in the KRas4B oncoprotein, which is mutated in 99% of PDAC cases [12]. Kras4B is a small GTPase, which belongs to the RAS protein subfamily, and it has essential functions in the control and regulation of normal cell proliferation. Human tumors almost always express mutated KRas4B proteins, from 90 to 99% of cases; specific mutations of this protein occur in codons 12, 13, or 61, which leaves the KRas4B protein constitutively active [11]. The active state of KRas4B proteins contributes significantly to develop the malignant phenotype, such as the deregulation of tumor cell growth, the evasion of programmed cell death, invasion, and angiogenesis [13]. There are three genes that code for RAS proteins in the mammalian genome: HRas, NRas, and KRas; four isoforms are obtained by alternative splicing: H-Ras, N-Ras, K-Ras4A, and K-Ras4B [14].

RAS subfamily proteins are also members of a broad class of proteins known as CAAX proteins [15] like this because the C-terminal end sequence has the CAAX amino acids (C: cysteine, A: aliphatic amino acid, and X: any amino acid), and this sequence is modified post-translationally in order to confer Ras protein affinity for the plasma membrane (for its subsequent activation). This process is regulated by three enzymes that work sequentially: first, the farnesyltransferase enzyme participates in the prenylation of the CAAX sequence; second, a protein called Ras-converting enzyme (RCE1) cleaves the last two amino acids of the CAAX sequence; third, a methyltransferase (ICMT) allows adding a methyl group to the carboxyl of the cysteine terminal to finally generate the mature RTP GTPase [16]. Farnesylation in the 185 cysteine terminal allows Ras proteins to increase their affinity for cell membranes and for many farnesyl group binding proteins that are analogous to RhoGDI transporters, such as phosphodiesterase 6 delta subunit (PDE6δ), which has been described as an indispensable molecule in the traffic of some GTPases of the Ras family [14, 17]. After the findings about the presence of KRas4B and its importance in the formation, maintenance, and progression of the most deadly neoplasms such as the PDAC [18, 19], studies have been conducted to discover and develop pharmacological inhibitors against oncogenic KRas4B. The approaches include: (a) finding small molecules that interact with KRas4B directly in order to prevent its activation [18, 19]; (b) finding enzyme inhibitors responsible for the post-translational modifications in order to prevent the transport of KRas4B to the plasma membrane; (c) finding compounds that inhibit the KRas4B downstream signaling pathway, as well as autophagy inhibitors and inhibitors of neoplastic cell metabolism [18, 19].

Despite the enormous prevalence of Kras4B mutations in pancreatic cancer, an efficient targeted treatment against aberrant signaling of this oncoprotein has not been found. It is known that pancreatic cancer cells with mutated Kras4B exhibit a phenomenon called "oncogene addiction", in which their survival becomes dependent on Kras4B signaling. Therefore, the inhibition of the Kras4B function promotes the inhibition of the viability of cancer cells; this eventually leads to cell death by apoptosis and the regression of the tumor [20, 21]. Therefore, it is necessary to find new strategies that allow us to inhibit the molecular mechanisms of activation and/or signaling of mutated Kras4B in pancreatic cancer. In this chapter, we describe new organic molecules that inhibit the dissociation of the heterodimeric molecular complex KRas4BG12C-D/PDE6δ; thus promoting that KRas4BG12C/D cannot bind to the plasma membrane, and consequently, it cannot be activated in pancreatic tumor cells.

2. Targeted drugs for the inhibition of KRas4B

The direct inhibition of KRas4B has been a difficult task. Sites susceptible to pharmacological interaction have been identified by means of bioinformatic programs; therefore, compounds such as SCH-53239 and its analogue SCH-54292, which presented low affinity with respect to KRas4B, have been identified. These compounds were designed to interact with the Switch II of KRas4B, competing with the GDP. These compounds have in their chemical structure a hydroxylamine, which is essential for their cytotoxic activity. These compounds present a high level of toxicity in murine models, so they are in the improvement phase [22]. In 2012, several research groups reported a compound called DCAI [22, 23], which interacts with KRas4B at the site located between the α2 helix and β4 loop; this compound was able to inhibit the interaction of SOS1 with KRas4B with an IC_{50} of 340 μM, having an EC_{50} of 15.8 μM; therefore, it is so far one of the compounds considered for the treatment of PDAC [22, 23]. Also, different research teams have been working on 11,000 analogues of the DCAI compound in silico, based on the nuclear magnetic resonance (NMR). One of the analogues called VU0460009, showed an IC_{50} of 240 μM; although the concentration of the mean inhibition decreased, this compound did not have a considerable effect in murine models, so it was not possible to consider it as a candidate for treatment of PDAC [22, 23]. In order to find an organic compound that was capable of inhibiting the activation of KRas4B, studies were conducted to direct a specific molecule to the location site of the KRas4BG12C mutation, which is the most frequent in lung cancer [22]. One of the compounds studied was the so-called SCH-54292 [12], which is capable of binding to the α2 and α3 helices of KRas4B. This compound showed activity only in the cell lines that present KRas4BG12C, and with this finding, the researchers have intended to identify and study the analogues of SCH-54292 with the greatest effect on cancer cell lines [12]. Another group of researchers created a GDP analogue called SML-8-73-1, which could covalently bind to the cysteine of KRas4BG12C without taking into account the affinity of GDP with its binding site in KRas4B. These compounds did not show the expected effect on lung cancer cell lines, so they are in the improvement phase [22]. In recent years, several research groups have been trying to selectively inhibit mutated KRas activation and signaling. One way to prevent the activation of KRas and, therefore, its effector pathways, is through allosteric inhibition. Consequently, several research groups have developed experimental models based on the *in silico* search for compounds that selectively bind and inhibit KRas. This strategy was carried out with an initial virtual coupling test of a library of compounds based on the reconstructed pocket structure of the switch I of RAS crystal, which resulted in an *in silico* coupling based on the pocket structure. The pocket consists of a hydrophilic part, which is composed of negatively charged residues such as Glu47, Asp48, and Asp 67, and a hydrophobic part, which consists of Leu66, Met77, and Tyr 81; on its surface, it is partially bordered by charged residues such as Lys15 and Asp67. These structural characteristics were used to establish a pharmacophore for the screening of charged residues, such as Asp67 (which corresponds to Asp57 of Ras), located in the lower center of the hydrophilic pocket in order to ensure the specificity of binding and energy. After the coupling analysis, compounds that *in vitro* effectively decreased the activation of Ras as well as its effectors were detected [21]. The development of small molecules that irreversibly bind to the oncogenic mutant KRasG12C allows the interruption of switch-1, and this alters the preference of native nucleotides in order to favor GDP over GTP and, consequently, this prevents its binding with the Raf effector. On the other hand, and using a similar strategy of *in silico* analysis and development of analogues with a favorable balance of ADME attributes (absorption, distribution, metabolism, and excretion), in vivo stability and specificity, in 2018, Janes and collaborators reported the design and characterization of switch-IIP inhibitors of KRasG12C with enhanced potency and pharmacological properties. Using tests based on liquid chromatography-tandem mass spectrometry (LC/MS-MS), compounds that covalently bound to Cys12 of K-Ras were measured directly and quantitatively. Pharmacological inhibition of KRasG12D with compound ARS-1620 suppressed the growth of cancer cells. ARS-1620 exhibited excellent oral bioavailability in mice and sufficient blood stability and, importantly, induces tumor regression through a specific mechanism of action.

Another strategy, proposed by Zeng and collaborators in 2017, is the possibility of designing compounds that incorporate elements of both the switch-IIP and the guanosine pharmacophores, or through the development of bivalent compounds that could recruit ligases to promote the degradation of RAS mediated by ubiquitination. The compounds were prepared with fluorophenyl and piperazinyl substituents and an electrophilic acrylamide warhead attached to the piperazine in order to effectively bind to KRasG12C. Subsequently, the 1_AM analogue was developed with an amino amide substituent and showed a more complete binding with KRas. In addition, 1_AM was compared with its serial head [1], and its properties were examined in H358 cells. The 1_AM inhibitor decreased levels of KRas bound to GTP by ~80% compared to the performance of inhibitor 1, and likewise the decrease of the ERK effector phosphorylated.

An interesting strategy, which has been recently addressed, is the blocking of the interaction of RAS with its effector Raf. A cyclic peptide called cyclosarin 9A5 blocked the RAS-RAF interaction. The amino acids present in cyclosarin such as nal, Fpa, Thr, norleucine (nle), and Trp are critical for binding with KRas. Cyclosarin 9A5 showed improved cell permeability and an affinity for KRas with an IC_{50} = 0.12 μM. Cyclosarin reduced the proliferation and induced cell death by apoptosis in tumor cells with mutated KRas [24].

Similarly, in 2019, MacCarthy and collaborators used a variety of computational approaches in order to describe four binding sites in K-Ras for allosteric ligands. The new inhibitors bind to the pocket p1 with submicromolar affinity and function primarily by directly inhibiting the interaction of KRas with its effector proteins. This potential inhibitor forms multiple favorable interactions with residues in the pocket p1 of nonmutated KRas (WT) and with residues of the mutants of K-RasG12D, G12C, and Q61H in the active state bound to GTP. In addition, the authors report that the inhibitor of KRas binding to its effectors decreases the levels of phosphorylation of ERK and cRAF in BHK cells that express the mutant of KRasG12D and G12V, which suggests the inhibition of KRas signaling through the MAPK pathway. However, the problem of allosteric KRas inhibitors that prevent interaction with their effectors is that they do not exhibit selectivity toward a particular RAS isoform or KRas WT vs. mutated KRas, which raises the toxicity problem in cells and therefore in healthy organs when they are used in vivo.

Another approach to inhibit the interaction of KRas with its effectors is the search for macromolecules that selectively bind to KRas at an allosteric lobe site that encompasses histidine 95 residue at the interface between the helix α3/loop 7/helix α4. Designed ankyrine repeat proteins (DARPins) K13 and K219 inhibit the interactions with the effectors and the nucleotide exchange of KRas. Similarly, K13 and K19 induce selective inhibition of the RAF/MEK/ERK signaling pathway in cells with the Kras4BG13D mutation but not in cells with other mutated isoforms such as HRasG12V and/or RAS WT. This suggests that K13 and K19 selectively inhibit the function of mutated KRas without affecting cancer cells with RAS WT; however, its toxicity in healthy cells has not been proven [25].

3. Targeted drugs for PDE6δ inhibition

Post-translational modifications are important for the recognition and transport of KRas4B to the plasma membrane; therefore, the study of molecules responsible for recognizing these post-translational modifications may be an important therapeutic target against PDAC [26]. One of the proteins responsible for recognizing the post-translational modification is phosphodiesterase 6δ (PDE6δ), which recognizes the farnesylation or geranyl-geranylation present in the cysteine of the CAAX motif of Kras4B protein [27]. A group of German researchers identified and evaluated the compound called Deltarasin, which interacts with PDE6δ, with a K_d of 38 nM, prevents the recognition of the post-translational modification present in KRas4B, arresting KRas4B in the cytosol, and consequently preventing its activation and tumor progression. This compound was named the first generation of PDE6δ inhibitors [26]. However, its evaluation in noncancerous pancreatic duct cell lines showed high cytotoxicity; this affected considerably the cell viability at low concentrations [28]. In 2016, the analogue of the compound Deltarasin (second generation of PDE6δ inhibitors) was reported, and it was called deltazinone. This analogue presented constant dissociation of K_d 38 nM to K_d 4 nM, thus showing to be a compound with better interaction energy than the analogue of first generation. Deltazinone showed cytotoxic effects on pancreatic cancer cell lines at a concentration of 24 μM, but it took about 8 h to have an anti-proliferative effect on pancreatic cancer cell lines. Conversely, Deltarasin, at a concentration of 5 μM showed the same effect in 1 hour. Considering these data, the first generation of PDE6δ inhibitors have a better performance than the ones from the second generation [29, 30]. In 2017, the third generation of specific PDE6δ inhibitors, which were called Deltasonamides, was reported. This new generation shows more interaction energy than the ones from the first generation and greater cytotoxic effects on pancreatic cancer cell lines at concentrations from 1 to 12 μM [31].

In early 2019, drugs based on triazoles arose. These compounds can be considered as the fourth generation of PDE6δ inhibitors since they used the structure of Deltarasin to be able to find the functional group with the highest interaction energy with PDE6δ. This fourth generation is still in *in vitro* studies in order to evaluate its cytotoxic effect [32]. At the beginning of 2020, the fifth generation of PDE6δ inhibitors, called Deltaflexin, arose; although they are analogues of Deltarasin, they do not have the same cytotoxic effects showed by the first generation of PDE6δ inhibitors [33].

4. Drugs capable of stabilizing the KRas4B/PDE6δ protein complex

The search for new targeted therapies aimed at trying to improve the quality of life of patients with pancreatic cancer has taken about 30 years; along this time, researchers have looked for compounds that can inhibit the signaling pathway of the KRas4B oncoprotein. One of the most important mechanisms for the activation of KRas4B is the transport from the cytosol toward the plasma membrane by the PDE6δ, which recognize the farnesyl group of KRas4B present at carboxyl terminal (**Figure 1a**). It was believed that KRas4B/PDE6δ was transported as a dimer, and it is now known that it forms a cluster of 6–12 proteins or 3–6 dimers (**Figure 1b**). Because of this, our work group looked for a plate of the heterodimer using the crystal of the heterodimeric complex of the cluster of 6 proteins (**Figure 1c**) in order to identify small organic molecules capable of stabilizing the interaction of the molecular complex KRas4B/PDE6δ with the purpose of avoiding the activation of KRas4B as well as its signaling pathway dependent of this oncoprotein. An exhaustive search was carried out in public chemical libraries of organic compounds

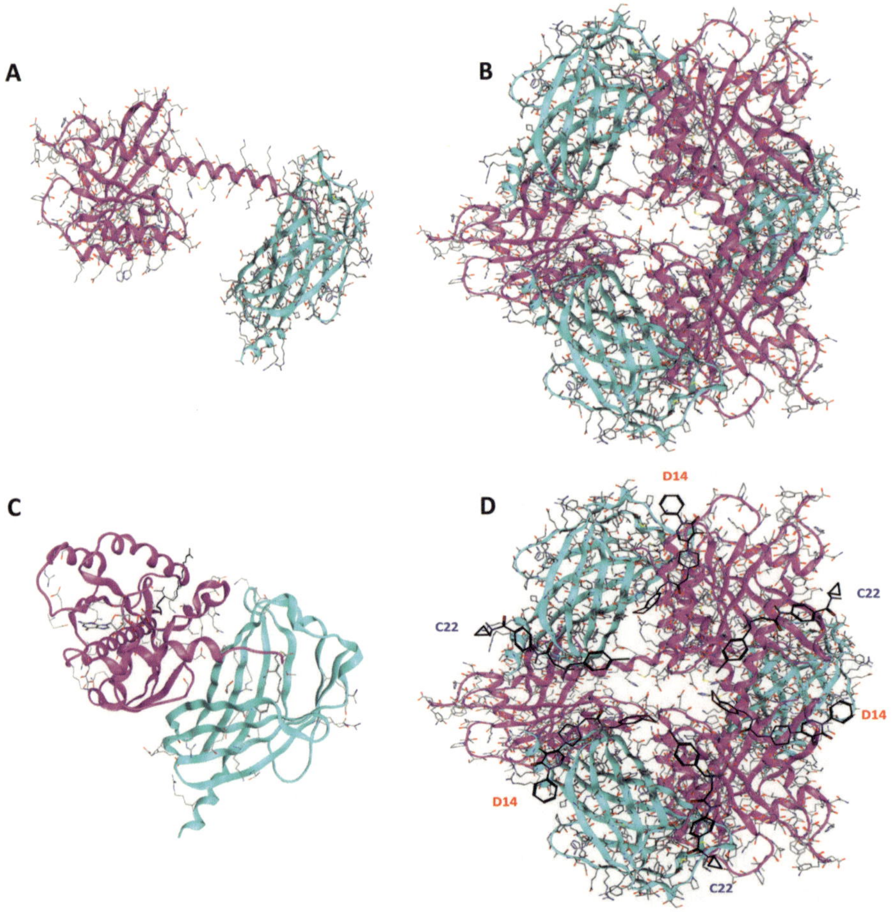

Figure 1.
Types of interactions between KRas4B/PDE6δ heterodimeric complex crystallized. (A) Interaction between K-Ras4B (pink) and PDE6δ (aqua) proteins. (B) Cluster formation among K-Ras4B/PDE6δ in multiheterodimeric molecular complexes crystallized. (C) Template of K-Ras4B/PDE6δ heterodimeric complex in a cluster used to docking and drug identification. (D) Molecular docking of D14 (N-[(2H-1,3-benzodioxol-5-yl)methyl]-2-[4-(5-chloro-6-oxo-1-phenyl-1,6-dihydropyridazin-4-yl)piperazin-1-yl]acetamide) and C22 (3-(2-{[1-(4 chlorophenyl)ethyl]amino}acetamido)-N-cyclopropylbenzamide) compounds and using a cluster of the heterodimeric K-Ras4B/PDE6δ molecular complexes.

with pharmacological potential, which could stabilize the KRas4B/PDE6δ complex. The identification of the compounds that had an *in silico* interaction with the complex, in addition these compounds was selected considering that they complied with the Lipinsky rule, which states that (1) the compounds should not have more than five hydrogen bridge donors; (2) they must not contain more than 10 hydrogen bridge acceptors; (3) they must have a molecular weight of less than 500 g/mol; (4) the compounds must have an octanol/water partition coefficient of less than five (log P < 5). Compounds identified as D14 and C22 showed different *in silico* interaction energies on the KRas4B/PDE6δ and K-Ras4BG12C/PDE6δ heterocomplex crystals; these interaction energies ranged from −143 to −162 ΔG [28].

An *in silico* analysis on the prediction of absorption using the ADME software made it possible to identify that compounds D14 and C22 have good absorption at the intestinal level and have low uptake by the permeability glycoprotein proteins that belong to the ABC transporter family. Their values are very low compared with the absorption of Gemcitabine and Deltarasin, which indicates that compounds D14 and C22 have a low chemoresistance when they are used as a treatment for pancreatic cancer cells (**Figure 2a**). Additionally, it was possible to observe a metabolism of compounds D14 and C22 by cytochromes P450 (CYP450), which indicated rapid liver metabolism and low toxicity since these compounds are coated by these enzymes (**Figure 2b**). Furthermore, it was observed that these compounds may have low toxicity compared to that obtained with the treatment of choice for pancreatic cancer such as Gemcitabine and with the PDE6δ Deltarasin inhibitor (**Figure 2c**).

Once identified that compounds D14 and C22 do not have toxic effects, we assessed the presence of KRas4B and PDE6d in pancreatic cancer cell lines by immunofluorescence using different cell lines with KRas4B (BxPC3), KRas4BG12D (PANC-1), and KRas4BG12C (MIA PaCa-2); we observed a greater presence of these proteins in the KRas PANC-1 and MIA PaCa-2-dependent cell lines (**Figure 3**). Having identified the cell lines with the highest presence of KRas4B and PDE6d, we treated them with a concentration of 200 μM of compounds D14 and C22 comparing their effect with hTERT-HPNE, which is a noncancerous cell line, and with 5 μM of Deltarasin (**Figure 4**). The results showed that compound D14 had a greater cytotoxic effect on the PANC-1 and MIA PaCa-2 cell lines, while compound C22 had a greater cytotoxic effect on the MIA PaCa-2 cell line. The comparison of these results with the effect obtained from Deltarasin, where the normal hTERT-HPNE cell line of pancreas was affected, suggested that our compounds do not have cytotoxicity in noncancerous cell lines.

Taking into account the results described above, we carried out Ras activation assays using the MIA PaCa-2 cell line. We obtained a dose response curve during 60 min, measuring Ras-GTP uptake by means of G-Lisa assays. Compounds D14 and C22 significantly decreased Ras activation over time; we obtained a 50% decrease in Ras activation at 60 min after treatment with the compounds (**Figure 5a**). As mentioned earlier during this chapter, the constitutive activation of KRas4B is essential for the development, progression, and maintenance of pancreatic cancer, and therefore, we performed subcutaneous xenograft tests by grafting 5 million cells of the MIA PaCa-2 cell line and administered via intraperitoneal 10 and 20 mg/kg of weight of compounds D14 and C22 for 15 days. The result was a 50% decrease in tumor growth in tumors treated with 20 mg/kg of weight of the two compounds, compared to the vehicle used as a control (**Figure 5b** and **c**).

Pancreatic ductal adenocarcinoma (PDAC) remains one of the leading causes of death by cancer, in addition to being one of the most aggressive types of cancer. The pancreatic cancer stem cell population (PCSCs) has been linked to this aggressiveness and poor prognosis. The cancer stem cell model proposes that tumor initiation,

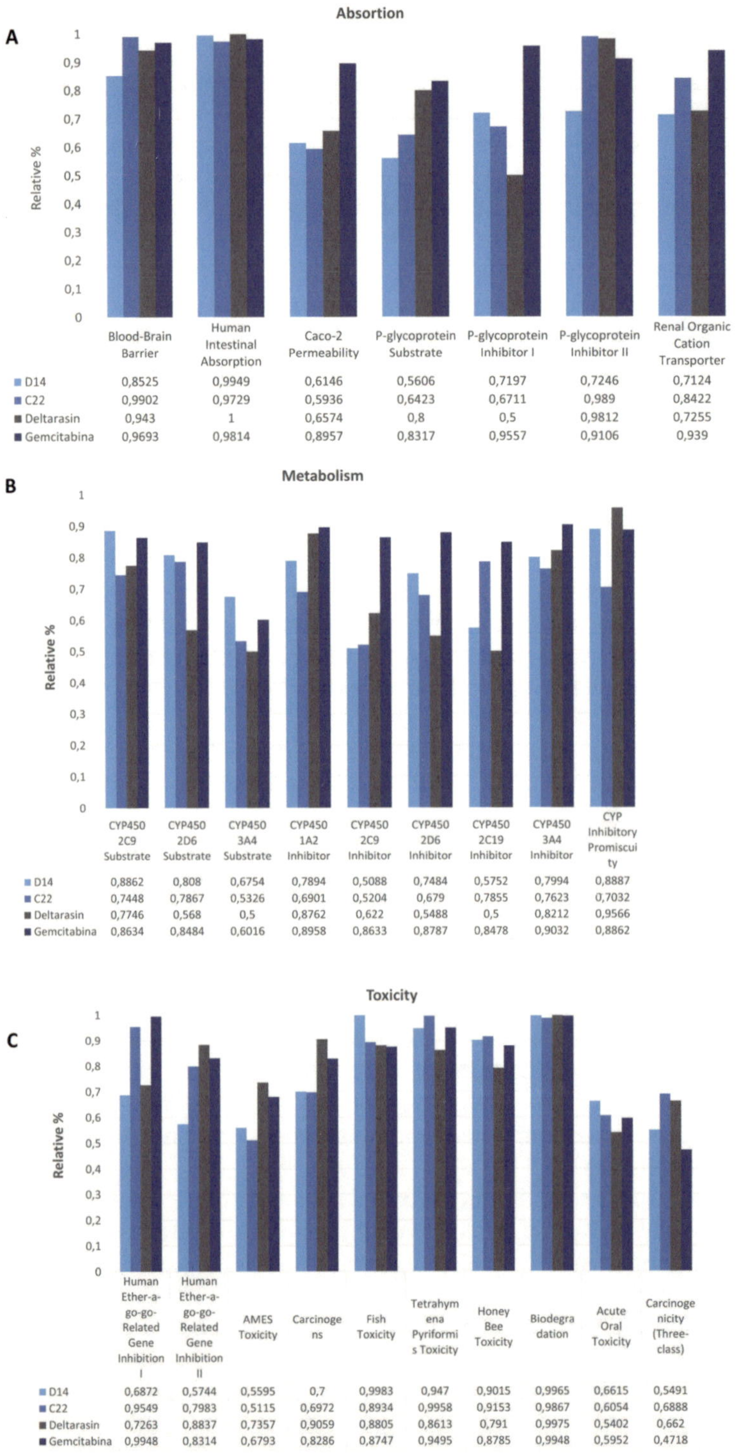

Figure 2.
Prediction of ADME processes of compounds D14 and C22. (A) Absorption of compounds D14 and C22 in epithelial barriers and their uptake by permeability glycoprotein proteins. (B) Metabolization of compounds D14 and C22 by means of cytochrome P450. (C) Toxicity of compounds D14 and C22.

maintenance, and growth are directed by the population of stem cancer cells (CSC) [34, 35], which have been identified in several types of cancer, *e.g.* breast, brain, head and neck, colon, and pancreas [36, 37]. CSCs are defined as those tumor cells

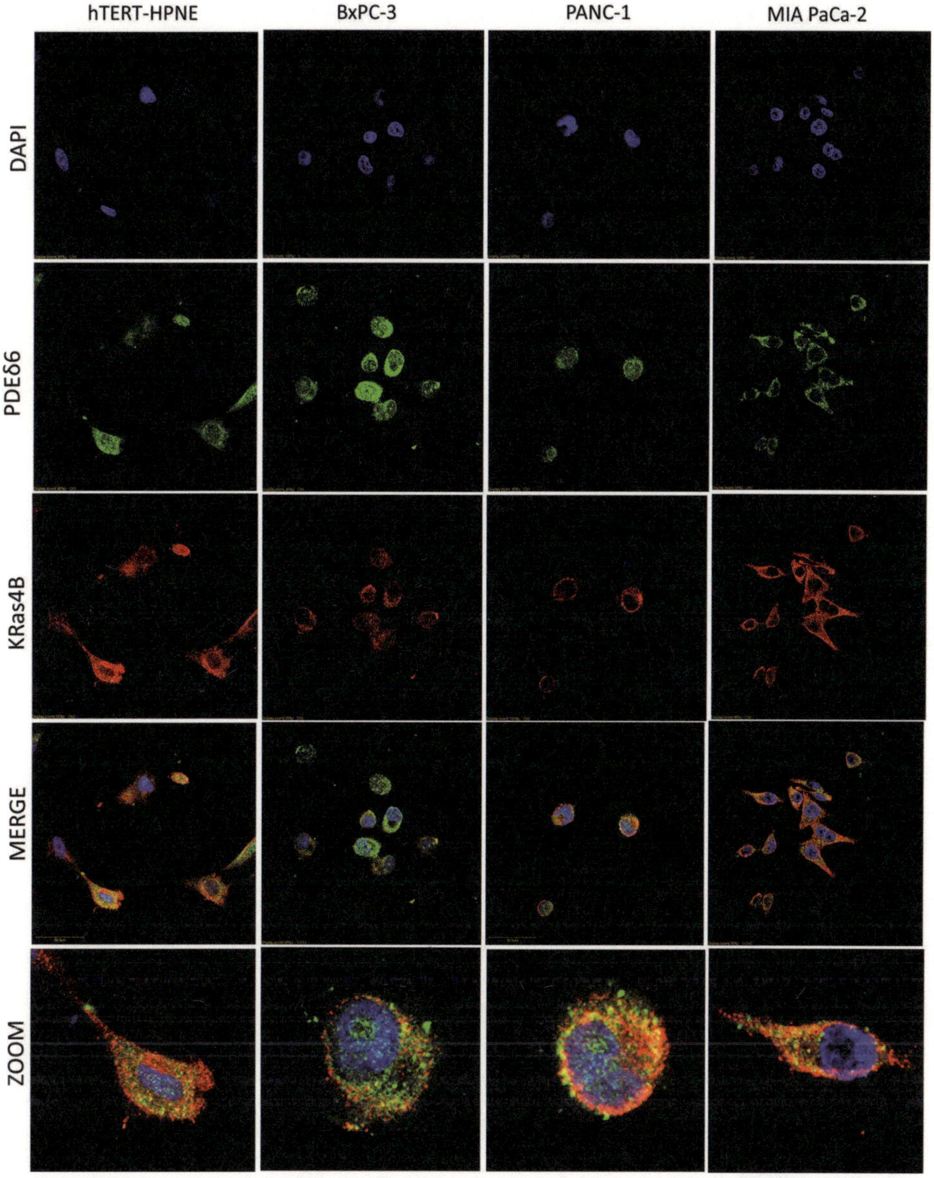

Figure 3.
KRas4B and PDE6δ are present in pancreatic cancer cell lines with different mutations in K-Ras. Images taken by confocal microscopy.

capable of self-renewal and production of heterogeneous lineages that comprise tumor volume [38]. In addition, several studies have reported evidence of the contribution of CSCs in resistance to conventional therapy, which causes metastasis and tumor recurrence [36, 39]. Different immunphenotypes have been reported for the identification of pancreatic cancer stem cells (PCSCs) [36, 37]. Due to the high fatality of PDAC, the importance of CSCs, and the participation of oncogenic KRas4B, we decided to evaluate the effect on the tumorigenicity of compounds D14 and C22 in CSC of PDAC; in this sense, cancer steam cells from BxPC3, PANC-1, and MIA PaCa-2 pancreatic cancer cell lines, as well as in the hTERT-HPNE non-cancerous cell line, were growing in nonadherent conditions, forming spheroids or pancreatospheres and selected with the immunophenotypes positive to CD44, CD24, and ESA markers, which indicates an enrichment of PCSC (**Figure 6**). These

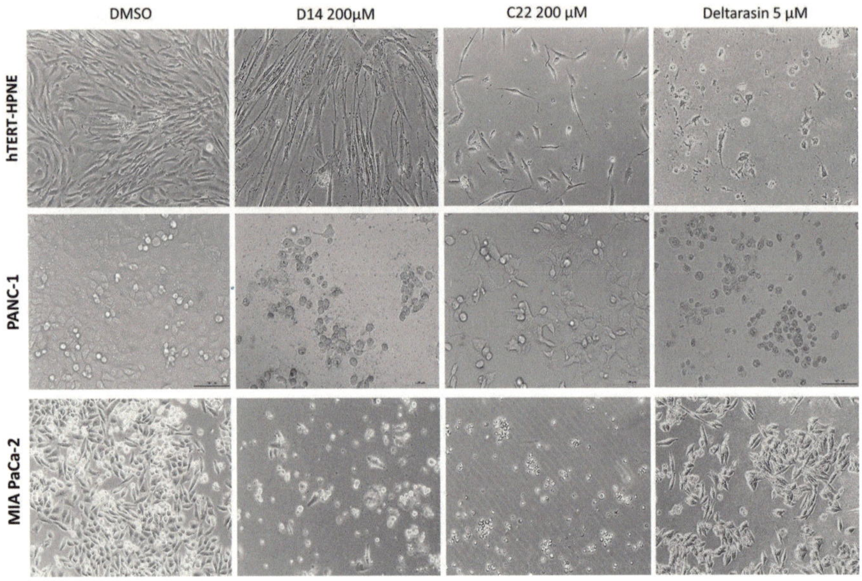

Figure 4.
Morphological visualization of hTERT-HPNE, PANC-1, and MIA PaCa-2 cell lines treated with compounds D14 and C22 at 200 μM compared with the effect of Deltarasin.

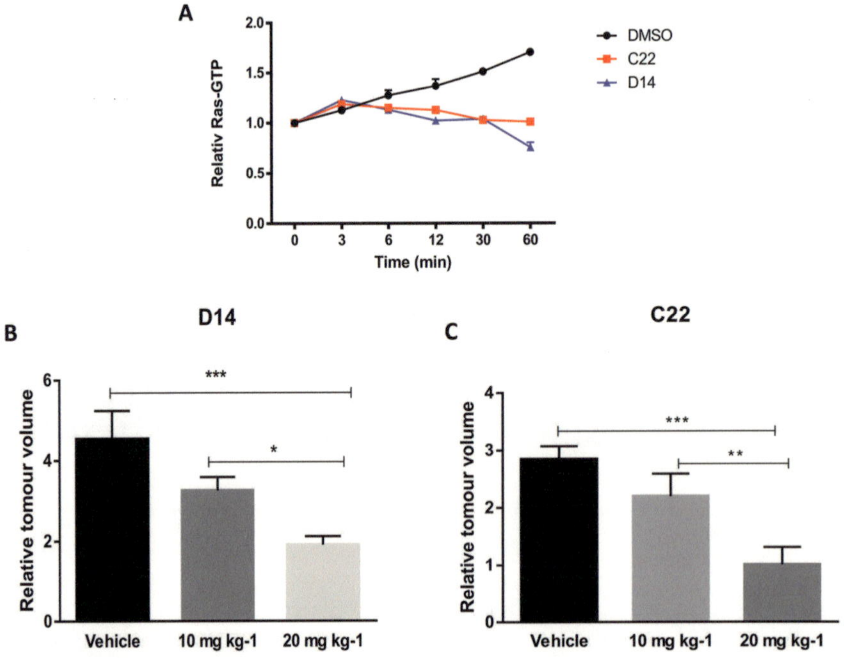

Figure 5.
Compounds D14 and C22 decrease the activation of Ras in the MIA PaCa-2 cell line promoting the decrease of tumor growth. (A) Ras activation decreases by more than 50% in the MIA PaCa-2 cell line treated with D14 and C22. (B) and (C) Compounds D14 and C22 decrease tumor growth in subcutaneous xenograft models, using 20 mg/kg and 10 mg/kg intraperitoneally for 15 days.

were treated with 49.65, 99.3, and 148.9 μM of compound D14, and with 494 nM of Gemcitabine. It was found that the treatment with compound D14 was able to break up the pancreatospheres formed by BxPC3 and MIA PaCa-2 more efficiently than the first-line treatment with Gemcitabine (**Figure 7**).

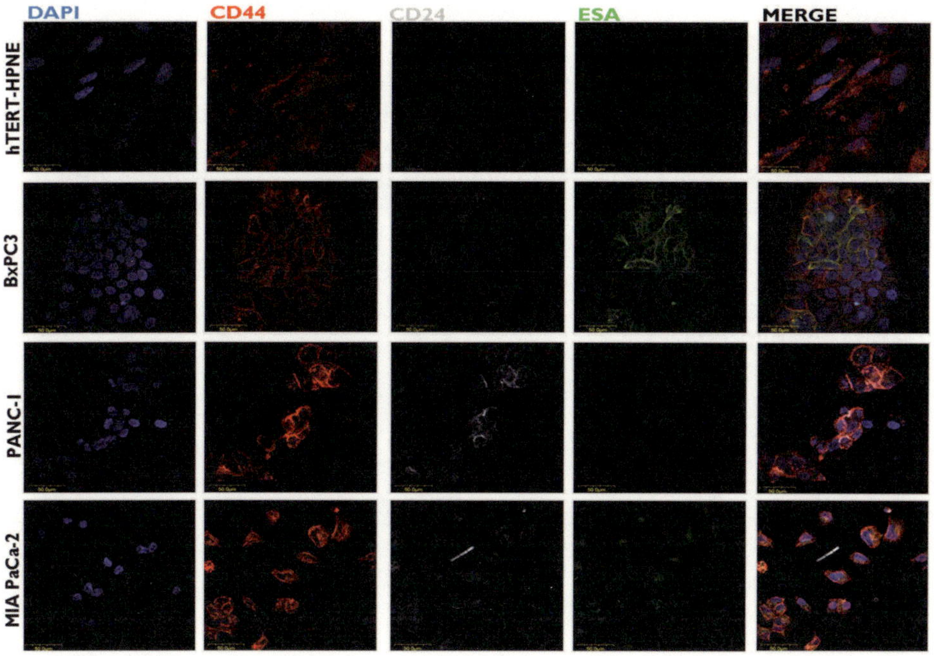

Figure 6.
CD44, CD24, and ESA immunophenotype in 3D cultures of BxPC3, PANC-1, and MIA PaCa-2. The expression of these markers is crucial for the identification of the cancerous trunk population.

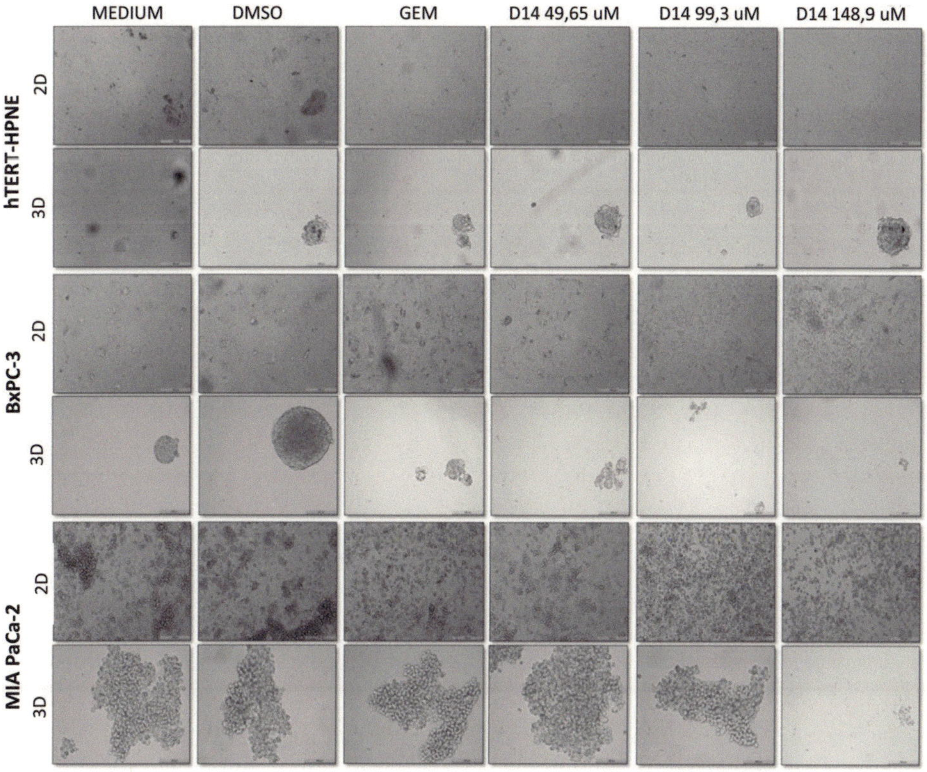

Figure 7.
Morphological visualization of the effect of compound D14 on the viability of BxPC3 and MIA PaCa-2 in 2D and 3D; the result is better than with Gemcitabine, which is the first-line treatment for PDAC.

5. Conclusion

The search for compounds that can stabilize the KRas4B/PDE6δ heterodimeric complex has provided a great pattern in the search for new and less toxic pharmacological alternatives for the treatment of pancreatic cancer and with fewer collateral effects due to their high specificity. Compounds D14 and C22 have shown great specific cytotoxic effects against pancreatic cancer cell lines as well as decreased tumor growth and, even better, in the possible reduction of the PCSC population. However, it is necessary to carry out additional experiments in order to identify the specific mechanisms of action of the cross-linking and stabilizing compounds of this protein multicomplex.

Author details

Paola Briseño-Díaz[1], Dora Emma Velez-Uriza[1], Pedro Cruz-Nova[1], Martiniano Bello Ramirez[2], Jose Correa-Basurto[2], Rosaura Hernandez-Rivas[1], Ma del Rocio Thompson Bonilla[3] and Miguel Ángel Vargas Mejía[1*]

1 Departamento de Biomedicina Molecular, Centro de Investigación y de Estudios Avanzados del Instituto Politécnico Nacional (CINVESTAV-I.P.N), Ciudad de México, Mexico

2 Laboratorio de Modelado Molecular y Diseño de Fármacos de la Escuela Superior de Medicina, Instituto Politécnico Nacional, México, Ciudad de México, Mexico

3 Investigación Biomédica y Traslacional, Laboratorio de Medicina Genómica, Hospital 1° de Octubre, ISSSTE, Ciudad de México, Mexico

*Address all correspondence to: mavargas@cinvestav.mx

References

[1] Abrams MJ, Rakszawski K, Vasekar M, Passero F, Abbas A, Jia Y, et al. Recent advances in pancreatic cancer: Updates and insights from the 2015 annual meeting of the American Society of Clinical Oncology. Therapeutic Advances in Gastroenterology. 2016;**9**(2):141-151

[2] Robbins SL, Kumar V, Cotran RS. Robbins and Cotran Pathologic Basis of Disease. 8th ed. Philadelphia, PA: Saunders/Elsevier; 2010

[3] Langley WC. Pancreatitis Research Advances. New York: Nova Biomedical Books; 2007

[4] Soreide K, Sund M. Epidemiological-molecular evidence of metabolic reprogramming on proliferation, autophagy and cell signaling in pancreas cancer. Cancer Letters. 2015;**356**(2 Pt A):281-288

[5] Qu CF, Li Y, Song YJ, Rizvi SMA, Raja C, Zhang D, et al. MUC1 expression in primary and metastatic pancreatic cancer cells for in vitro treatment by 213Bi-C595 radioimmunoconjugate. Cancer Research. 2004;**0007-0920**(04): 2086-2093

[6] Lahdaoui F, Delpu Y, Vincent A, Renaud F, Messager M, Duchene B, et al. miR-219-1-3p is a negative regulator of the mucin MUC4 expression and is a tumor suppressor in pancreatic cancer. Oncogene. 2015;**34**(6):780-788

[7] Adsay NV, Merati K, Andea A, Sarkar F, et al. The dichotomy in the preinvasive neoplasia to invasive carcinoma sequence in the pancreas: Differential expression of MUC1 and MUC2 supports the existence of two separate pathways of carcinogenesis. Modern Pathology. 2002;**15**(10):1087-1095

[8] Tinder TL, Subramani DB, Basu GD, Bradley JM, Schettini J, Million A, et al. MUC1 enhances tumor progression and contributes toward immunosuppression in a mouse model of spontaneous pancreatic adenocarcinoma. Journal of Immunology. 2008;**181**(5):3116-3125

[9] Gillen S, Schuster T, Meyer Zum Buschenfelde C, Friess H, Kleeff J. Preoperative/neoadjuvant therapy in pancreatic cancer: A systematic review and meta-analysis of response and resection percentages. PLoS Medicine. 2010;**7**(4):e1000267

[10] Hezel AF, Kimmelman AC, Stanger BZ, Bardeesy N, Depinho RA. Genetics and biology of pancreatic ductal adenocarcinoma. Genes & Development. 2006;**20**(10):1218-1249

[11] Bardeesy N, DePinho RA. Pancreatic cancer biology and genetics. Nature Reviews Cancer. 2002;**2**(12):897-909

[12] Zeitouni D, Pylayeva-Gupta Y, Der CJ, Bryant KL. KRAS mutant pancreatic Cancer: No lone path to an effective treatment. Cancers (Basel). 2016;**8**(4):45

[13] Castellano E, Downward J. Role of RAS in the regulation of PI 3-kinase. Current Topics in Microbiology and Immunology. 2010;**346**:143-169

[14] Ahearn IM, Haigis K, Bar-Sagi D, Philips MR. Regulating the regulator: Post-translational modification of RAS. Nature Reviews. Molecular Cell Biology. 2011;**13**(1):39-51

[15] Boguski MS, McCormick F. Proteins regulating Ras and its relatives. Nature. 1993;**366**:643

[16] Wang Y, Kaiser CE, Frett B, Li HY. Targeting mutant KRAS for anticancer therapeutics: A review of novel small molecule modulators. Journal of Medicinal Chemistry. 2013;**56**(13):5219-5230

[17] Dharmaiah S, Bindu L, Tran TH, Gillette WK, et al. Structural basis of recognition of farnesylated and methylated KRAS4b by PDEdelta. Proceedings of the National Academy of Sciences of the United States of America. 2016;**113**(44):E6766-E6775

[18] Cox AD, Der CJ. Ras history: The saga continues. Small GTPases. 2010;**1**(1):2-27

[19] Buhrman G, O'Connor C, Zerbe B, Kearney BM, Napoleon R, Kovrigina EA, et al. Analysis of binding site hot spots on the surface of Ras GTPase. Journal of Molecular Biology. 2011;**413**(4):773-789

[20] Park D, Shakya R, Koivisto C, Pitarresi JR, et al. Murine models for familial pancreatic cancer: Histopathology, latency and drug sensitivity among cancers of Palb2, Brca1 and Brca2 mutant mouse strains. PLoS One. 2019;**14**(12):e0226714

[21] Shima F, Yoshikawa Y, Ye M, Araki M, et al. In silico discovery of small-molecule Ras inhibitors that display antitumor activity by blocking the Ras-effector interaction. Proceedings of the National Academy of Sciences of the United States of America. 2013;**110**(20):8182-8187

[22] Cox AD, Fesik SW, Kimmelman AC, Luo J, Der CJ. Drugging the undruggable RAS: Mission possible? Nature Reviews Drug Discovery. 2014;**13**(11):828-851

[23] Ostrem JM, Peters U, Sos ML, Wells JA, Shokat KM. K-Ras(G12C) inhibitors allosterically control GTP affinity and effector interactions. Nature. 2013;**503**(7477):548-551

[24] Upadhyaya P, Qian Z, Selner NG, Clippinger SR, Wu Z, Briesewitz R, et al. Inhibition of Ras signaling by blocking Ras-effector interactions with cyclic peptides. Angewandte Chemie (International Ed. in English). 2015;**54**(26):7602-7606

[25] Bery N, Legg S, Debreczeni J, Breed J, et al. KRAS-specific inhibition using a DARPin binding to a site in the allosteric lobe. Nature Communications. 2019;**10**(1):2607

[26] Zimmermann G, Papke B, Ismail S, et al. Small molecule inhibition of the KRAS-PDEdelta interaction impairs oncogenic KRAS signalling. Nature. 2013;**497**(7451):638-642

[27] Scott AJ, Lieu CH, Messersmith WA. Therapeutic approaches to RAS mutation. Cancer Journal. 2016;**22**(3):165-174

[28] Casique-Aguirre D, Briseno-Diaz P, Garcia-Gutierrez P, et al. KRas4B-PDE6delta complex stabilization by small molecules obtained by virtual screening affects Ras signaling in pancreatic cancer. BMC Cancer. 2018;**18**(1):1299

[29] Chuang HC, Huang PH, Kulp SK, Chen CS. Pharmacological strategies to target oncogenic KRAS signaling in pancreatic cancer. Pharmacological Research. 2017;**117**:370-376

[30] Simanshu DK, Nissley DV, McCormick F. RAS proteins and their regulators in human disease. Cell. 2017;**170**(1):17-33

[31] Martin-Gago P, Fansa EK, Klein CH, et al. A PDE6delta-KRas inhibitor chemotype with up to seven H-bonds and picomolar affinity that prevents efficient inhibitor release by Arl2. Angewandte Chemie (International Ed. in English). 2017;**56**(9):2423-2428

[32] Chen D, Chen Y, Lian F, Chen L, Li Y, Cao D, et al. Fragment-based drug discovery of triazole inhibitors to block PDEdelta-RAS protein-protein interaction. European Journal of Medicinal Chemistry. 2019;**163**:597-609

[33] Siddiqui FA, Alam C, Rosenqvist P, Ora M, Sabt A, Manoharan GB, et al.

PDE6D inhibitors with a new design principle selectively block K-Ras activity. ACS Omega. 2020;**5**(1):832-842

[34] Liu S, Dontu G, Wicha MS. Mammary stem cells, self-renewal pathways, and carcinogenesis. Breast Cancer Research. 2005;**7**(3):86-95

[35] Reya T, Morrison SJ, Clarke MF, Weissman IL. Stem cells, cancer, and cancer stem cells. Nature. 2001;**414**(6859):105-111

[36] Hermann PC, Bhaskar S, Cioffi M, Heeschen C. Cancer stem cells in solid tumors. Seminars in Cancer Biology. 2010;**20**(2):77-84

[37] Li C, Heidt DG, Dalerba P, Burant CF, Zhang L, Adsay V, et al. Identification of pancreatic cancer stem cells. Cancer Research. 2007;**67**(3):1030-1037

[38] Clarke MF, Dick JE, Dirks PB, Eaves CJ, Jamieson CH, Jones DL, et al. Cancer stem cells—Perspectives on current status and future directions: AACR workshop on cancer stem cells. Cancer Research. 2006;**66**(19):9339-9344

[39] Miranda-Lorenzo I, Dorado J, Lonardo E, Alcala S, Serrano AG, Clausell-Tormos J, et al. Intracellular autofluorescence: A biomarker for epithelial cancer stem cells. Nature Methods. 2014;**11**(11):1161-1169

Chapter 4

Computer Assistance in the Minimally Invasive Ablation Treatment of Pancreatic Cancer

Benjamin Eigl, Andreas Andreou, Matthias Peterhans, Stefan Weber and Beat Gloor

Abstract

The insertion of ablation needles towards pancreatic tumors demands excellent anatomical knowledge and interdisciplinary skills from the medical professional. While the placement of a single needle next to the structures at risk surrounding the pancreas is considered a challenging task, irreversible electroporation requires multiple needles to be placed in parallel at a specific location. Minimally invasive procedures complicate the already ambitious procedure, yet the ablation method bears potential to increase the overall survival for patients with locally advanced pancreatic cancer. Current studies require more clinical evidence regarding the efficacy of irreversible electroporation in pancreatic cancer by means of randomized controlled, multicenter trials. However, the ablation treatment is currently applied in expert centers only, which is due to the complex task of the needle placement. Computer-assisted surgery has shown its potential in different fields of applications to improve the targeting of diseased tissue and the confidence of the medical professional. The application of computer-assisted needle navigation for pancreatic cancer ablation holds the prospect to make the procedure more reproducible and safer.

Keywords: pancreatic cancer, needle guidance, irreversible electroporation, Computer-assisted surgery

1. Introduction

Pancreatic cancer is one of the most aggressive types of cancer in the abdominal cavity with poor survival rates below 10% [1]. The reasons for the poor prognosis range from late detection of the cancer, vascular invasion, and difficult access due to the surrounding structures at risk. Attributable to the late detection, 80% of patients are not eligible for resection as they are diagnosed with locally advanced (30%), or metastatic pancreatic cancer (50%) [2]. Patients with locally advanced pancreatic cancer can benefit from alternatives such as radiotherapy, high-intensity focused ultrasound (HIFU), or ablation as a complementary treatment. Over the last decade, local ablative techniques have been used more frequently in patients without metastatic disease. Several techniques, all of which were primarily introduced in order to ablate liver metastases are in clinical use. Radiofrequency or microwave ablation, the two most widely established techniques, use thermal energy. However, high temperatures not only destroy tumor tissue but also increase morbidity if applied too close to structures such as bile duct, portal vein, superior mesenteric vein, celiac artery, or superior mesenteric artery, which all run in close proximity to the pancreas [3–5]. On the other hand, irreversible electroporation (IRE) leads to cell death by using high-voltage electrical pulses without destroying vascular collagen [6]. IRE, in contrast to thermal ablative techniques, always requires at least two needles, and metallic implants and cardiac arrhythmias are contraindications for this technique [6]. Possible morbidity arises either from needle tract injuries (bleeding, local infection due to intestinal puncture) or from energy application-associated thrombosis or necrotic tissue leading again to infection.

Local ablative techniques are generally used in the context of a multimodal treatment. Preoperative chemotherapy has been established in the most recent years for the multimodal treatment of borderline resectable and locally advanced pancreatic cancer to increase resectability [7]. Neoadjuvant chemoradiation has also been increasingly performed with favorable long-term outcomes [8]. However, response to these treatments cannot be evaluated adequately using radiologic criteria so far, thus directing decision-making regarding resection [9]. Similarly, IRE for pancreatic cancer has been facing the same problems, lacking reliable radiologic and clinical markers for the detection of response. Nevertheless, current studies have indicated that the antitumoral efficacy of IRE may be identified using immunological parameters supporting the oncological benefits of IRE, additional to the electroporative effects of this ablative method on tumor cells [10, 11].

Neoadjuvant treatment for borderline resectable or locally advanced pancreatic cancer may allow resection in up to 78% of selected patients [12]. In this case, R0 resection status has been previously described as essential to reduce local and systemic recurrence and prolong survival [13]. However, due to local extension of tumor to involve vascular structures, R0 resection is more difficult to be achieved in patients with advanced disease and positive resection margins have been frequently been underestimated [14]. Therefore, in advanced disease, multimodal treatment concepts including induction therapy, followed by resection and concomitant IRE at the surgical margins have been proposed [15]. Several studies have shown the safety and feasibility of margin accentuation with intraoperative IRE during resection for borderline resectable and locally advanced pancreatic cancer. According to this concept, intraoperative IRE before complete transection could accentuate the negative-margin dissection of the retroperitoneal margin and its surrounding perivascular soft tissue as well as the perineural and mesenteric tissue adjacent to critical vascular structures [16, 17].

Additionally, current studies have even provided most promising results in terms of reduced local and distant progression, and superior overall survival when pancreatic resection and IRE are combined [16, 17]. Careful selection of patients eligible for this strategy, together with modern systemic therapy regimens, may increase resectability and improve oncological outcomes in the near future [18].

In patients with borderline resectable and locally advanced pancreatic cancer, IRE was also identified as a valuable tool to offer consolidative disease control and symptom relief such as pain control and to support eradiation of the malignant lesion [19]. However, only few studies have evaluated the quality of life following IRE for pancreatic cancer [20]. In a recent study, 84 patients undergoing IRE for locally advanced pancreatic cancer were enrolled. Quality of life assessment indicated that IRE therapy does not impair the quality of life in the short term. Adverse post-interventional events such as increased insomnia and constipation at 3 months and diarrhea at 6 months after IRE are most probably related to other clinical factors such as chemotherapy-associated toxicity. Therefore, IRE is not expected to adversely affect long-term quality of life in this patient cohort [21]. Further studies are required to examine quality of life following IRE in the long term.

The latest numbers on published pancreatic IRE cases investigated by Moris et al. [22] counted a total of 498 treatments and accentuate the lack of clinical evidence as an indicator for low numbers in pancreatic IRE treatments compared to other fields of application. While the procedures were either conducted percutaneously (n = 232) or open (n = 262), the laparoscopic approach (n = 4) played only a minor role [22].

IRE application requires the user to place the needles within a certain distance and angle to each other [23]. This makes the use of the ablation technique very difficult, especially when navigating the needles close to structures at risk. With respect to the laparoscopic needle placement, the long needles and decreased field of view add additional complexity to this task.

2. Navigate the pancreas

The workflow for pancreatic IRE treatments is divided into a preoperative planning and intraoperative navigation phase.

2.1 Preoperative needle planning

Tomographic images are acquired to identify the structures at risk in proximity to the tumor. These structures include vessels, bile ducts, and organs as visualized in **Figure 1**.

To assess suitable patients for the IRE treatment, patients are screened to determine possible access windows and the needle configuration depending on the treatment approach [24]. In addition, 3D reconstructions derived from the original images enhance the spatial understanding during the planning of the trajectories.

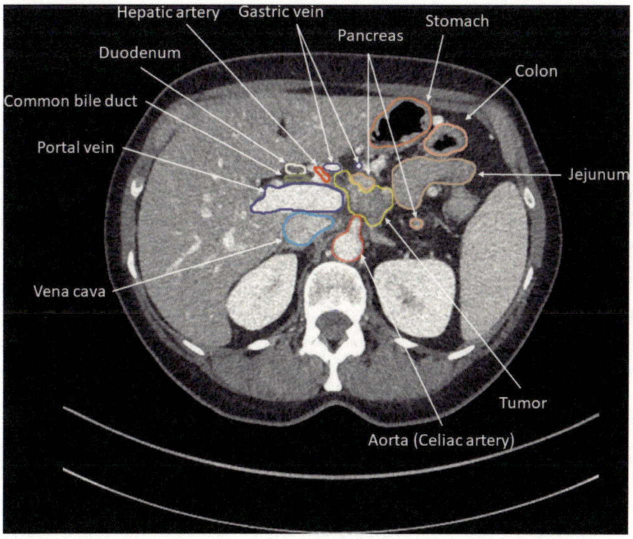

Figure 1.
Axial computed tomography image of a patient with LAPC where the tumor encapsulates the celiac artery.

However, information regarding the preoperative IRE planning phase remains sparse in current literature.

2.2 Intraoperative needle placement

While the surgical (open or laparoscopic) approach provides advantages to mobilize the structures at risk to gain a better access window for the needles, the review of all eligible studies until August 2018 identified a morbidity of 36% for the surgical approach (89/247) compared to 24.3% for the percutaneous IRE approach (56/230) [22].

Atraumatic needle placement is key for a successful treatment outcome; thus, the needles need to be monitored with computed tomography (CT), magnetic resonance imaging (MRI), fluoroscopy, or with live ultrasound (US) depending on the treatment approach. As of today, there is no comparative study investigating CT vs. US-guided IRE needle placement. Both modalities may be used to check for proper needle placement [19, 25, 26]. However, since preoperative planning is typically conducted on CT images, it may be considered as the primary modality for guiding needle placement during the percutaneous intervention. The main disadvantage of increased radiation can be considerably reduced by complementing computer-assisted navigation, as will be discussed later [27]. In addition, CT-guided procedures are less dependent on the experience of the user and offer the possibility to check immediately for post-interventional complications such as bleeding or thrombosis [27, 28].

The flexibility of the needles represents an additional challenge to keep the needles on track during the insertion. Dedicated hardware tools provide additional support to guide the needle to the specific location by reducing bending artifacts. The most basic form of needle guidance is the usage of the needle spacer provided by AngioDynamics (Latham, New York) to achieve the desired interelectrode distance, yet it does not prevent the needle from bending during the insertion [29]. Martin et al. [30, 31] emphasize the usage of a needle guide attached to the biplanar US probe for more precise needle placement and to keep the needle in the ultrasound plane. However, this approach limits the spatial freedom of the ultrasound transducer due to the static properties of the guide and aggravates the monitoring of structures at risk.

3. The doctor's opinion

To elaborate on the necessity of dedicated planning and navigation assistance, we conducted a questionnaire with eight medical doctors (MDs). The study population consisted of MDs with specialty in HPB surgery (n = 7) and surgical oncology (1) active in USA (1), India (1) Turkey (1), Germany (1), Austria (1), and Switzerland (3). The MDs performed between 30 and 120 pancreatic surgeries annually (average value of 70 surgeries per year). The yearly number of IREs was situated between 0 and 20 treatments with an average number of 4.5. All questioned doctors performed the preoperative planning of IRE cases solely on tomographic images and occasionally in combination with reconstructed 3D models. Due to the complex anatomy with varying patient-specific structures at risk, all MDs argue in favor of a preoperative IRE planning tool, which makes use of imaging data in combination with reconstructed 3D models to verify the feasibility of needle configurations. Most of the pancreas specialists see a need for minimally invasive pancreas IRE (87.5%) as well as for intraoperative needle navigation (100%) (illustrated in **Figure 2**) [32].

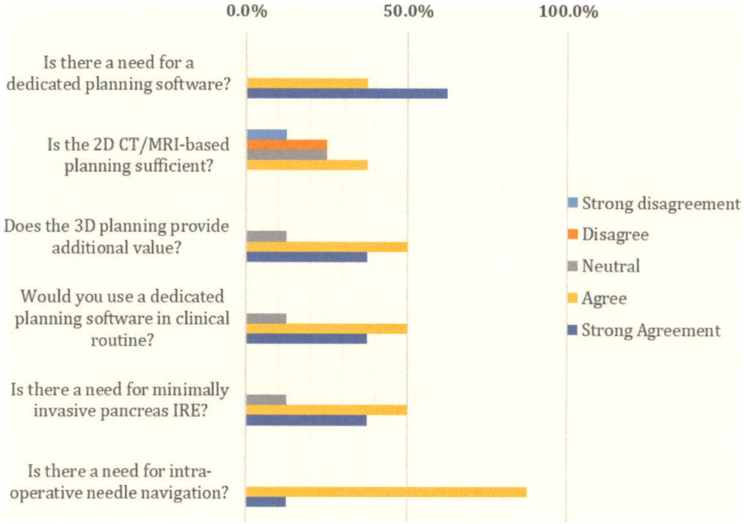

Figure 2.
Result from questionnaire where the need for dedicated tools is highlighted to assist the clinician in the perioperative procedure.

4. Computer-assisted needle guidance

Computer-assisted surgery (also known as stereotactic surgery) is established in fields like orthopedics and neurosurgery and emerged from "being just around the corner" to clinical routine of abdominal surgery over the recent decade [33]. When it comes to needle guidance, Beerman et al. [34] have reported the experiences from 1000 consecutive cases using computer-assisted image-guidance in liver ablations. The key message of this study is the necessity of navigation solutions with respect to reproducibility in percutaneous, laparoscopic, and open interventions [34]. Another report investigating the accuracy between guided and manual probe placement shows a significant advantage for the guided approach [35]. Martin et al. [36] discuss the advantages of computer assistance in the placement of single needles during a liver phantom study demonstrating that 95% of the participants were able to hit the center of the tumor using the computer-assisted approach compared to 65% with ultrasound (US) only.

The system used in the above studies was designed by CAScination (Bern, Switzerland) and provides guidance for interventional and surgical liver procedures (see **Figure 3**).

With regard to minimally invasive applications the system discriminates between the percutaneous and laparoscopic approach in the following aspects:

4.1 Percutaneous ablation

The navigation system supports the clinician during percutaneous ablation, which is performed in the intervention suite using computed tomography (CT) or cone-beam CT (CBCT) imaging. The patient is under general anesthesia with respiratory motion control and positioned on a vacuum mattress. Retroreflective single markers are attached to the patient's skin using a dedicated marker template. The single markers are detectable by the optical tracking camera and in the tomographic images and build the foundation for virtual to physical space registration. Furthermore, their spatial position is used for monitoring of patient movement throughout the procedure. The needle trajectories are then planned, navigated, and verified using CT images, with the possibility of planning IRE needle configurations (**Figure 4**).

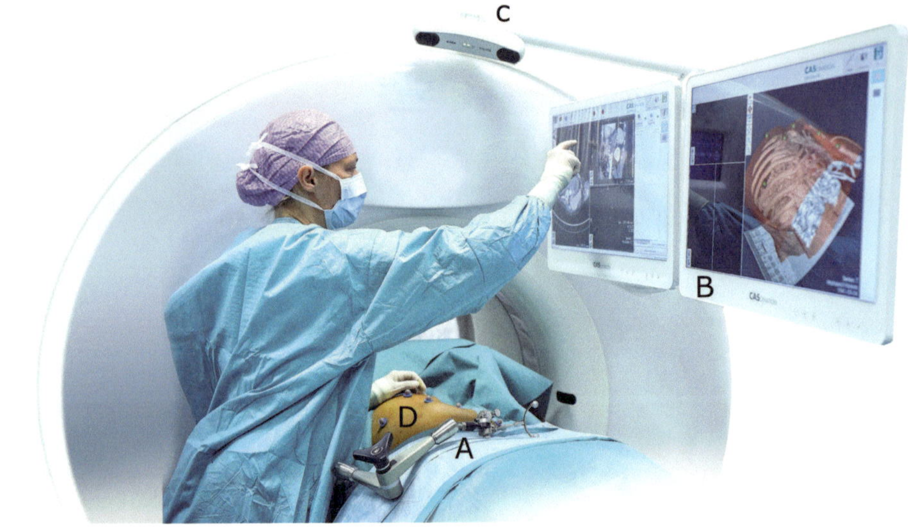

Figure 3.
Setup for percutaneous needle insertion. Aiming device (A), touch monitors (B), optical tracking camera (C), patient markers (D).

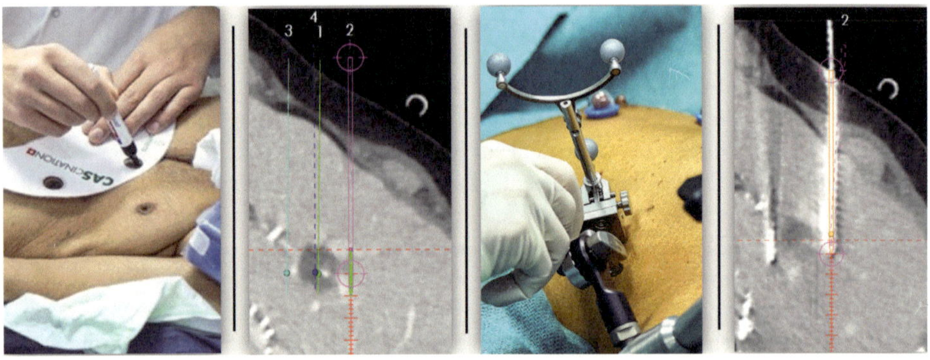

Figure 4.
Percutaneous workflow from left to right: Patient marker attachment, CT-based IRE trajectory planning, positioning of aiming device, and needle placement control.

For the initial planning image, contrast-enhanced CT is the preferred choice to achieve a good discrimination between the structures of interest. To further enhance the planning procedure, a preoperative MRI image can be fused with the intraoperative image data to visualize structures not traceable in the intraoperative CT.

Lachenmayer et al. [37] retrospectively analyzed the system in 174 percutaneous ablations of hepatocellular carcinoma (HCC) and reported a median lateral error of 3.2 (0.2–14.1) mm. They concluded that percutaneous, computer-assisted needle navigation is safe and efficient for treatment of HCC. Beyer et al. [38, 39] evaluated the system against manual, CT-fluoroscopically guided probe placement for IRE of liver tumors. The CAScination guidance (n = 10) was compared against manual guidance (n = 10) and they reported a significant decrease in planning time (55 vs. 104 min, $P < 0.001$) and radiation exposure. The procedural accuracy, measured as the deviation of the IRE electrodes with respect to a defined reference electrode, was significantly higher for the navigated approach (2.2 vs. 3.3 mm mean deviation, $P < 0.001$) [39].

4.2 Laparoscopic ablation

The system for laparoscopic needle navigation relies on a surface landmark registration in which distinct points on the organ surface are sampled with tracked instruments and matched with the corresponding points from available patient image data. These data include preoperative CT images with optional 3D reconstructions from structures of interest. Guidance is achieved by tracking of the ablation needle using retroreflective markers attached to the hand piece (**Figure 5**).

A major drawback for the surface landmark-based registration approach is organ deformation due to pneumoperitoneum, which downgrades navigation accuracy on preoperative image data. Intraoperative CT imaging would help to reduce deformation artifacts; however, this requires the availability of a hybrid OR [40]. Prevost et al. [41] investigated the laparoscopic guidance solution for liver resection and ablation in 10 cases with the main conclusion being that the navigation system enhances the explorative phase, yet the registration accuracy was not sufficient for reliable tool navigation. Stillström et al. [42] pioneered in the application of computer assistance in laparoscopic pancreas IRE. They reported the feasibility of image-guided navigation in the operating theater even though the system was mainly used for orientation purposes.

4.3 Needle guidance

The CAScination system distinguishes between two approaches for needle guidance, namely active and passive guidance. The active guidance (freehand approach) makes use of instrument calibration to determine the needle tip with respect to the marker shield attached to the hand piece of the needle, whereas passive guidance makes use of a tracked mechanical arm (aiming device approach) which is pre-calibrated due to known geometric properties. While the former provides the advantage of visualizing the needle tip during the insertion to obtain an active depth control, it is affected by errors resulting from the calibration and needle bending. The latter is not affected by the calibration error and reduces the bending artifacts by means of brackets guiding the needle along the oriented path. During needle insertion, the lateral deviation from the original plan is of high significance as it may require needle repositioning. Wallach et al. [43] compared the two approaches during a phantom study with 25 needle punctures on a nonrigid phantom. The resulting lateral error of the needle to the defined target was found to be significantly lower with the aiming device (2.3 ± 1.3 mm vs. 4.2 ± 2.0 mm) [43].

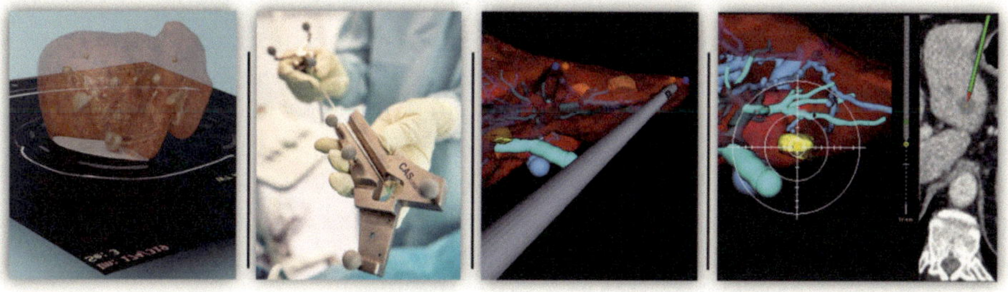

Figure 5.
Laparoscopic workflow from left to right: preoperative image segmentation, optical instrument calibration, landmark-based registration, targeting with active depth control.

4.4 Alternative navigation solutions

There are a number of navigation solutions for abdominal organs on the market. These devices share the same fundamental functional principles and provide a different range of functionalities, which can be used in the setting of IRE on the pancreas. Given the high accuracy requirements and the complexity in needles placement relative to a number of risk structures, we deem functionality for multi-needle planning as well as accurate needle guidance as mandatory requirements for navigated IRE on the pancreas. The following paragraphs present different available navigation solutions and evaluate them with respect to these two requirements.

The IMACTIS® CT (Imactis SAS, La Tronche, France) solution is designed for percutaneous interventions using CT imaging and electromagnetic instrument tracking. The device was applied on different target organs and available literature includes an assessment of needle positioning accuracy and time requirements in a prospective randomized trial. The median Euclidean error [interquartile range] using the computer-assisted approach was found to be 4.1 mm [2.7–9.1 mm] compared to 8.9 mm [4.9–15.1 mm] for the non-navigated group for a total of 120 patients [44]. This shows that IMACTIS® CT has the potential to reach sufficient accuracy for IRE needle placement. Its shortcoming with respect to the application of pancreatic IRE lies in the fact that the device has no functionality for needle planning and multi-needle treatments.

The MAXIO (Perfint Healthcare, Florence, Oregon, USA) is used in CT-guided, percutaneous interventions and includes a robotic arm for needle placement. The device comprises a planning software supporting single- as well as multi-needle planning for different needle types. Beyer et al. [38] investigated the MAXIO with respect to procedural accuracy in a retrospective study of 40 cases of liver IRE conducted by an experienced interventional radiologist. Out of these, 19 were conducted using manual needle placement under CT fluoroscopy guidance and 21 with guidance of the robotic system. To calculate the procedural accuracy, an oblique slice was placed at the needle tip closest to the tumor with the normal pointing along the needle direction. Each needle tip was successively projected on the slice translated 3 cm from the tip toward the hand piece to calculate the distance to the needle center. The resulting accuracy was significantly improved when comparing the robotic approach to freehand needle placements (2.2 vs. 3.1 mm) [38].

The navigation system Explorer (Pathfinder) is designed for needle guidance in open liver surgery and is based on optical instrument tracking (same functional principle as CAS-One for the laparoscopic use case). A study by Bond et al. [45] investigated needle guidance accuracy and required time in a randomized controlled trial of IRE for pancreatic cancer. The application of the Explorer device decreased time for needle placement from 20 to 11 min while reaching an accuracy of 3.4 mm in relative spacing between the needles. The accuracy of needle placement with respect to the target anatomy is expected to be lower as the publication reports average fiducial registration errors of 10.8 mm. The authors conclude that the main benefit of the navigated approach is the increase of the surgeon's confidence to localize the needle using stereotactic navigation. The image to physical space registration is seen as the biggest obstacle to achieve a reliable overlay between the preoperative plan and the intraoperative scene.

Further guidance solutions for pancreatic IRE potentially include the use of ultrasound fusion devices such as those used in percutaneous ablation treatment on the liver. While providing needle guidance under real-time feedback, there are no devices providing multi-needle planning functionality together with ultrasound-based needle navigation. To our knowledge, there are no reports on the usage of ultrasound-fusion and navigation devices in the setting of pancreatic IRE.

5. Computer-assisted pancreas navigation

Existing computer-assisted navigation solutions address the needs of the pancreatic MDs to some extent, yet there remains room for improvement. The application of IRE as a treatment for pancreatic cancer bears additional challenges, which are partially covered by existing solutions:

- The IRE needle configuration is dependent on the tumor size. The optimal spacing between two IRE probes shall be situated between 1.5 and 2.5 cm to achieve a successful treatment outcome [23].
- Multiple structures at risk surrounding the pancreas require the probes to be planned and placed according to safety criteria to reduce insertion related complications [22, 25].
- The flexible IRE needles increase the risk of deformation during the insertion process.
- A homogeneous ablation field along the active zone of the IRE needles is dependent on the parallelism of the inserted needles [46].

Low usage numbers of stereotactic needle guidance in the pancreatic use case highlights that not all problems have yet been addressed to support the complete perioperative procedure. A study recently published by He et al. [47] demonstrated the feasibility of robot-assisted percutaneous IRE treatment of pancreatic head cancer in 9 cases. With respect to spatial accuracy, the stereotactic percutaneous navigation outperformed the stereotactic laparoscopic navigation in existing reporting. Therefore, stereotactic percutaneous needle guidance can be seen as the foundation to achieve reliable and reproducible navigation results. Yet, it only constructs one part of a dedicated computer-assisted pancreatic IRE workflow.

5.1 IRE planning tool

Preoperative image data are essential to generate a safe and feasible ablation plan with an optimal needle configuration to treat the tumor. We developed a dedicated preoperative planning tool, which makes use of CT/MRI image data in combination with 3D reconstructions to simulate IRE needle configurations. The tool allows the MD to define target and entry positions on multiplanar reconstructions (MPR) of the tomographic images with the possibility to select different needle configurations (layout and spacing). Under consideration of IRE-related constraints (spacing and parallelism), the trajectories can be optimized to cover the region of interest. The segmentations are conducted by a radiologist using dedicated software and can be tailored upon the type of intervention. Unlike for the open approach, preoperative segmentations for a percutaneous approach could include structures like the stomach, colon, or liver as well. This information is beneficial for the determination of the access window and to evaluate risk structures in the vicinity of the needles.

The planning tool was evaluated in the course of a clinical study of IRE in a laparotomy setting at the local hospital (Inselspital, Bern, Switzerland). **Figure 6** demonstrates the application of the planning tool to 1 out of 10 cases. During the surgery, the decision was to place the needles according to plan # 1 as the superior mesenteric vein was not mobilizable enough to obtain a window for the inferior right needle in #2. The 3D planning tool proved beneficial in both the preoperative

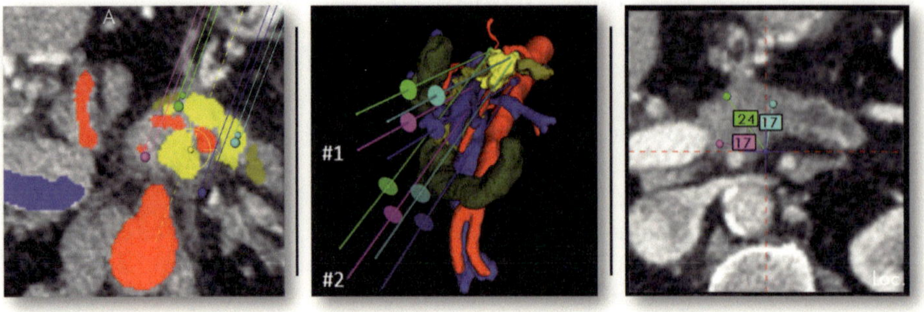

Figure 6.
Preoperative plan on axial plane with segmentation overlay (left). Two IRE configurations with 3D reconstructions (middle). Image plane at needle tip in direction of the trajectory to visualize distances between the needles in millimeter (right).

as well as intraoperative phase as it increased the MDs spatial understanding during the generation of the ablation plan.

5.2 Aiming for parallelism

To transfer the predefined ablation plan from theory to practice, a navigation system can take remedial action. Visual guidance information provided by the navigation system aids the clinician to position the ablation needle relative to the defined path. The computer-assisted navigation solutions proved to be advantageous for IRE needle guidance in terms of procedural accuracy compared to the manual, CT-fluoroscopically guided approach [38, 39]. Whereas these navigation systems make use of a mechanical guide, navigation systems such as the IMACTIS® CT require the user to actively align and insert the needle. This might cause a challenge for less experienced clinicians in needle guidance. We have therefore compared the two computer-assisted navigation approaches discussed in Section 4.3 by means of a phantom study with a similar setup as in [43]. Firstly, the needle was actively tracked (freehand approach), and secondly the mechanical arm (aiming device approach) was used. Seven participants were requested to place three needles (17 g, 15 cm) using each approach around a tumor encompassing the celiac artery in an artificial, flexible phantom. Three trajectories were predefined on the navigation system and each user received an instructional training. The calibration procedure for the freehand approach was conducted upfront to minimize the calibration error. The starting sequence was randomized, the needle control scan was conducted with a mobile C-arm, and the validation again conducted with the CAScination system by means of image to image fusion.

The mean lateral error for the aiming-device approach (2.4 ± 0.7 mm) was found to be similar compared to the lateral error (2.3 ± 1.3 mm) obtained in [43]. The error for the freehand approach resulted in a larger mean error (6.7 ± 1.7 mm) compared to the results from [43] (4.2 ± 2.0 mm), which can be explained by the larger group of participants with varying experience in manual needle placement. Parallelism of the needles for both approaches was calculated according to the method used in [38] where an oblique slice was placed at the needle closest to the tumor with the normal pointing along the needle direction. Each needle tip was successively projected on the plane translated 3 cm from the tip toward the handpiece to calculate the distance to the needle center. With a total of 14 samples per approach, the resulting mean Euclidean error was significantly lower for the aiming device than for the freehand approach (1.5 ± 0.7 mm versus 2.4 ± 1.1 mm) with a p-value of 0.014 (see **Figure 7**). However,

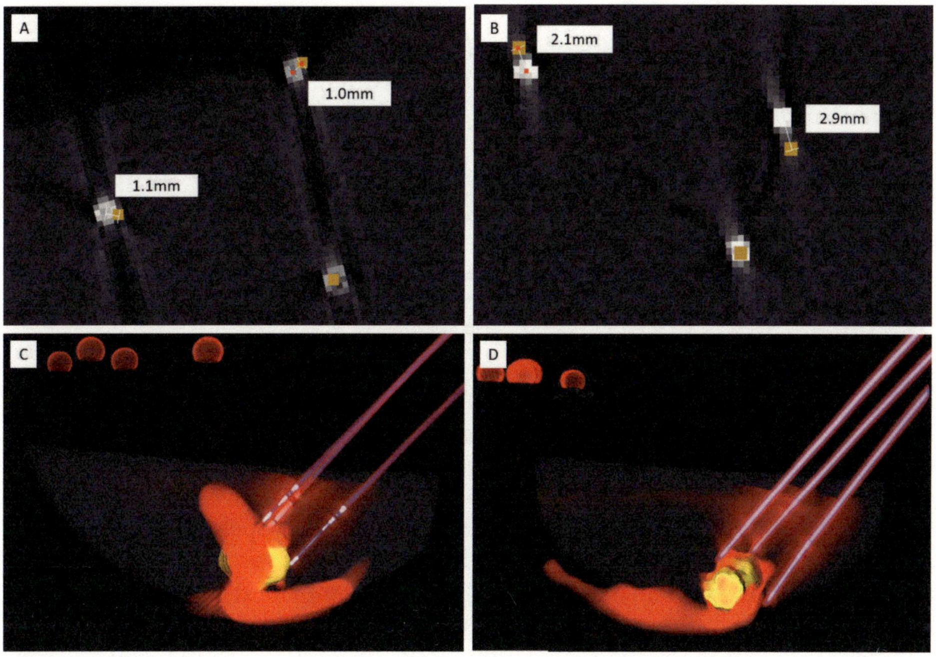

Figure 7.
Comparison of aiming device versus freehand for a specific participant. The top row visualizes the calculation of the Euclidean error between the aiming device (A) and freehand (B) approach. Volume rendering from control CT of aiming device (C) and freehand (D) guidance highlights the bending of the needle in the freehand approach.

these results should not be compared with the findings by Beyer et al. [38, 39] due to the setup of the studies (phantom vs. in vivo), yet their reported decrease of the error using the computer-assisted navigation goes along with the findings by our group.

6. Future directions of IRE in pancreatic cancer

Given the severity and decreased overall survival of patients diagnosed with locally advanced pancreatic cancer, there is a driving need for treatment alternatives to conventional chemo/radiation therapy. The minimally invasive application of IRE shows potential regarding an increase of the progression-free survival time and quality of life [48]. However, these interventions require highly experienced medical professionals as needles need to be navigated close to multiple structures at risk. Computer assistance plays a major role in all types of procedures where spatial accuracy needs to be delivered in order to achieve a successful treatment outcome. As mentioned in Morris et al. [22] there is a need for multicenter, randomized, prospective trials to determine the efficacy of IRE treatment in the pancreatic use case. To conduct IRE treatments on the pancreas, computer assistance holds the potential to standardize the workflow and to enable highly accurate needle placement independent on outstanding multidisciplinary skills, which are typically found in high expert centers.

6.1 Patient screening

The evaluation of suitable patients for IRE is a crucial step to achieve a positive treatment outcome. The Miami Protocol lists patients' criteria including among others the performance status, lesion size, and access path [24]. An important criterion is stated by the access path, which requires an excellent radiological understanding due to the difficulty of planning multiple trajectories solely on tomographic images. This coincides with the opinions of the MDs who consider conventional 2D planning to be insufficient. A dedicated planning tool would enhance the preoperative procedure as multiple access paths can be planned relative to the patient's anatomy and structures at risk better identified. This requires precise anatomical segmentations from the radiological department, which is, especially for the pancreatic use case, a time-consuming task.

6.2 Artificial intelligence-driven segmentation

To plan multiple trajectories, especially in a percutaneous fashion, multiple organs surrounding the pancreas need to be considered. To obtain a good spatial understanding of the acquired tomographic images, 3D representations from the structures of interest help in the decision-making process. Where time may be sufficiently available in the preoperative phase, it is a valuable asset during the intraoperative phase. Therefore, a compromise between accuracy and processing time must be chosen to enable 3D reconstruction from intraoperative tomographic images. Deep learning-based segmentation has shown its potential in multiple fields including medical imaging tasks [49]. Segmentation of the pancreas is seen as a challenging task due to the dependency on good delineation of the organ to its adjacent structures in the abdominal cavity [50]. To segment the complete range of structure needed for pancreas IRE planning, Roth et al. [51] describe a multi-scale pyramid of 3D fully convolutional network. The reported network was trained and validated using 377 clinical CT datasets with annotated organs and vessels. The performance of the system was measured by means of the DICE score, which represents the similarity between the automatic segmentations from CT images not used for training and their manual annotations. The network was able to achieve a Dice score close to 90% on average, which holds promising aspects for automatic, intraoperative segmentation [51].

6.3 Automatic trajectory optimization

Based on the patient-specific data, automatic trajectories can be computed according to permitted access paths while securing a specific distance to structures at risk [52]. The optimization for the IRE use case would further depend on the needle configuration, interelectrode spacing, and parallelism constraints.

6.4 Ablation zone prediction

The application of IRE lacks the possibility of ablation validation as, in contrast to thermal ablation, the ablation zone cannot be monitored in real time. Therefore, the clinician must fully rely on the ablation zone prediction from the manufacturer, which is based on mathematical and ex vivo models. However, ultrasound elastography has shown potential to distinct ablated tissue from normal liver parenchyma with respect to tissue stiffness, which peaked 4 hours post-ablation [53]. Based on the ultrasound characteristics at 2 hours post-ablation in combination with histopathology findings, Bhutiani et al. [54] have shown the mismatch of current models with in vivo-generated ablation volumes in porcine liver and spleen.

6.5 From theory to practice

The placement of needles according to the defined trajectories is seen as a challenging task, especially for medical professionals who are not versatile in the art of needle insertion. Therefore, navigation solutions are of great interest to empower these clinicians to conduct safe procedures with IRE in the pancreas. Needle navigation by means of software and hardware guidance is best applicable to improve the spatial accuracy and to spare structures at risk. Especially the aiming device has shown its value in the reduction of needle bending for inexperienced users. Further improvement toward parallel insertion of the electrodes is required since this is, next to the interelectrode spacing, an important aspect to achieve a homogeneous ablation volume.

7. Conclusion

Minimally invasive ablation treatment of locally advanced pancreatic cancer is a promising, yet challenging task. The application of the IRE as a treatment addition to conventional chemotherapy with optional radiotherapy has the potential to increase the overall survival, which needs further investigation upon its efficacy by means of randomized-controlled, multicenter studies. The percutaneous application of IRE demands a sophisticated workflow from preoperative screening of suitable patients to intraoperative implementation of the predefined ablation plan. Computer-assisted surgery systems can aid the clinician during these steps with dedicated software and hardware tools to achieve reproducible and effective treatments.

Acknowledgements

Benjamin Eigl was supported by the European Union's Horizon 2020 Research and Innovation programme under grant agreement no. 722068.

Conflict of interest

Benjamin Eigl is employed as a PhD student at CAScination, with his salary covered by the European Union's Horizon 2020 Research and Innovation programme. Matthias Peterhans is the CSO and cofounder of CAScination. Stefan Weber is CEO and cofounder of CAScination.

Author details

Benjamin Eigl[1,2*], Andreas Andreou[3], Matthias Peterhans[2], Stefan Weber[2] and Beat Gloor[3]

1 ARTORG Center for Biomedical Engineering Research, Bern, Switzerland

2 CAScination AG, Bern, Switzerland

3 Department of Visceral Surgery and Medicine, Inselspital, University of Bern, Bern, Switzerland

*Address all correspondence to: benjamin.eigl@artorg.unibe.ch

References

[1] Siegel RL, Miller KD, Jemal A. Cancer statistics, 2017. CA: A Cancer Journal for Clinicians. 2017;**67**(1):7-30. Available from: http://onlinelibrary.wiley.com/doi/10.3322/caac.21387/abstract

[2] O'Kane GM, Knox JJ. Locally advanced pancreatic cancer: An emerging entity. Current Problems in Cancer. 2018;**42**(1):12-25. Available from: https://linkinghub.elsevier.com/retrieve/pii/S014702721730106X

[3] Saccomandi P, Lapergola A, Longo F, Schena E, Quero G. Thermal ablation of pancreatic cancer: A systematic literature review of clinical practice and pre-clinical studies. International Journal of Hyperthermia. 2018;**35**(1):398-418. DOI: 10.1080/02656736.2018.1506165

[4] Pezzilli R, Ricci C, Serra C, Casadei R, Monari F, D'Ambra M, et al. The problems of radiofrequency ablation as an approach for advanced unresectable ductal pancreatic carcinoma. Cancer. 2010;**2**:1419-1431

[5] Wu Y, Tang Z, Fang H, Gao S, Chen J, Wang Y, et al. High operative risk of cool-tip radiofrequency ablation for unresectable pancreatic head cancer 1. Journal of Surgical Oncology. 2006;**94**(5):392-395

[6] Holzgang M, Eigl B, Erdem S, Gloor B, Worni M. Irreversible Electroporation in Pancreatic Cancer. IntechOpen; 2018. DOI: 10.5772/intechopen.75737

[7] Versteijne E, Vogel JA, Besselink MG, Busch ORC, Wilmink JW, Daams JG, et al. Meta-analysis comparing upfront surgery with neoadjuvant treatment in patients with resectable or borderline resectable pancreatic cancer. British Journal of Surgery. 2018;**105**:946-958

[8] Jang JY, Han Y, Lee H, Kim SW, Kwon W, Lee KH, et al. Oncological benefits of neoadjuvant chemoradiation with gemcitabine versus upfront surgery in patients with borderline resectable pancreatic cancer: A prospective, randomized, open-label, multicenter phase 2/3 trial. Annals of Surgery. 2018;**268**(2):215-222

[9] Katz MHG, Fleming JB, Bhosale P, Varadhachary G, Lee JE, Wolff R, et al. Response of borderline resectable pancreatic cancer to neoadjuvant therapy is not reflected by radiographic indicators. Cancer. 2012;**118**(23):5749-5756

[10] Scheffer HJ, Stam AGM, Geboers B, Vroomen LGPH, Ruarus A, de Bruijn B, et al. Irreversible electroporation of locally advanced pancreatic cancer transiently alleviates immune suppression and creates a window for antitumor T cell activation. Oncoimmunology. 2019;**8**(11):1652532

[11] Pandit H, Hong YK, Li Y, Rostas J, Pulliam Z, Li SP, et al. Evaluating the regulatory immunomodulation effect of irreversible electroporation (IRE) in pancreatic adenocarcinoma. Annals of Surgical Oncology. 2019;**26**(3):800-806

[12] Michelakos T, Pergolini I, Del Castillo CF, Honselmann KC, Cai L, Deshpande V, et al. Predictors of resectability and survival in patients with borderline and locally advanced pancreatic cancer who underwent neoadjuvant treatment with FOLFIRINOX. Annals of Surgery. 2019;**269**(4):733-740

[13] Maeda S, Moore AM, Yohanathan L, Hata T, Truty MJ, Smoot RL, et al. Impact of resection margin status on survival in pancreatic cancer patients after neoadjuvant treatment and pancreatoduodenectomy. Surgery (United States). 2020;**167**(5):803-811

[14] Esposito I, Kleeff J, Bergmann F, Reiser C, Herpel E, Friess H, et al. Most pancreatic cancer resections are R1 resections. Annals of Surgical Oncology. 2008;**15**(6):1651-1660

[15] Martin RCG, McFarland K, Ellis S, Velanovich V. Irreversible electroporation in locally advanced pancreatic cancer: Potential improved overall survival. Annals of Surgical Oncology. 2013;**20**(S3):443-449. DOI: 10.1245/s10434-012-2736-1

[16] Kwon D, McFarland K, Velanovich V, Martin RCG. Borderline and locally advanced pancreatic adenocarcinoma margin accentuation with intraoperative irreversible electroporation. In: Surgery. Mosby Inc.; 2014. pp. 910-922

[17] Marsanic P, Mellano A, Sottile A, De Simone M. Irreversible electroporation as treatment of locally advanced and as margin accentuation in borderline resectable pancreatic adenocarcinoma. Medical & Biological Engineering & Computing. 2017;**55**(7):1123-1127

[18] Conroy T, Hammel P, Hebbar M, Ben Abdelghani M, Wei AC, Raoul JL, et al. FOLFIRINOX or gemcitabine as adjuvant therapy for pancreatic cancer. New England Journal of Medicine. 2018:2395-2406

[19] Martin RCG, Kwon D, Chalikonda S, Sellers M, Kotz E, Scoggins C, et al. Treatment of 200 locally advanced (Stage III) pancreatic adenocarcinoma patients with irreversible electroporation safety and efficacy. Annals of Surgery. 2015:486-492

[20] Braucci A, Niglio A, Molino C. Pancreatic cancer: Does irreversible electroporation improve the quality of life and the survival in local advanced pancreatic adenocarcinoma? Report of a pilot case. Pancreatology. 2013;**13**(3):S45

[21] Field W, Rostas JW, Martin RCG. Quality of life assessment for patients undergoing irreversible electroporation (IRE) for treatment of locally advanced pancreatic cancer (LAPC). American Journal of Surgery. 2019;**218**(3):571-578

[22] Moris D, Machairas N, Tsilimigras DI, Prodromidou A, Ejaz A, Weiss M, et al. Systematic review of surgical and percutaneous irreversible electroporation in the treatment of locally advanced pancreatic cancer. Annals of Surgical Oncology. 2019;**26**(6):1657-1668. DOI: 10.1245/s10434-019-07261-7

[23] Narayanan G. Irreversible electroporation. Seminars in Interventional Radiology. 2015;**32**(4):349-355. Available from: http://www.ncbi.nlm.nih.gov/pubmed/26622097

[24] Venkat S, Hosein PJ, Narayanan G. Percutaneous approach to irreversible electroporation of the pancreas: Miami protocol. Techniques in Vascular and Interventional Radiology. 2015;**18**(3):153-158

[25] Narayanan G, Hosein PJ, Arora G, Barbery KJ, Froud T, Livingstone AS, et al. Percutaneous irreversible electroporation for downstaging and control of unresectable pancreatic adenocarcinoma. Journal of Vascular and Interventional Radiology. 2012;**23**(12):1613-1621. Available from: http://linkinghub.elsevier.com/retrieve/pii/S1051044312009591

[26] Mansson C, Bergenfeldt M, Brahmstaedt R, Karlson B-M, Nygren P, Nilsson A. Safety and preliminary efficacy of ultrasound-guided percutaneous irreversible electroporation for treatment of localized pancreatic cancer. Anticancer Research. 2014 Jan;**34**(1):289-293

[27] Sánchez Y, Anvari A, Samir AE, Arellano RS, Prabhakar AM, Uppot RN. Navigational guidance and ablation

planning tools for interventional radiology. Current Problems in Diagnostic Radiology. 2017;**46**:225-233

[28] Ruarus AH, Vroomen LGPH, Geboers B, van Veldhuisen E, Puijk RS, Nieuwenhuizen S, et al. Percutaneous irreversible electroporation in locally advanced and recurrent pancreatic cancer (PANFIRE-2): A multicenter, prospective, single-arm, phase II study. Radiology. 2019:191109. DOI: 10.1148/radiol.2019191109

[29] AngioDynamics. NanoKnife™ User Manual Version 2.2.0. User Manual United States ed. Latham, New York: AngioDynamics; 2010. p. 91

[30] Martin RCG. Irreversible electroporation of locally advanced pancreatic head adenocarcinoma. Journal of Gastrointestinal Surgery. 2013;**17**(10):1850-1856. DOI: 10.1007/s11605-013-2309-z

[31] Martin RCG II. Irreversible electroporation of locally advanced pancreatic neck/body adenocarcinoma. Journal of Gastrointestinal Oncology. 2015;**6**(3):329-335. Available from: http://www.ncbi.nlm.nih.gov/pubmed/26029461

[32] Eigl B, Peterhans M, Weber S, Gloor B, Worni M. Evaluation of a 3D Planning Tool for Irreversible Electroporation Treatment in Pancreatic Cancer. Turin: Society for Medical Innovation and Technology; 2017. p. 1

[33] Kenngott HG, Wagner M, Nickel F, Wekerle AL, Preukschas A, Apitz M, et al. Computer-assisted abdominal surgery: new technologies. Langenbeck's Archives of Surgery. 2015;**400**(3):273-281. DOI: 10.1007/s00423-015-1289-8

[34] Beermann M, Lindeberg J, Engstrand J, Galmén K, Karlgren S, Stillström D, et al. 1000 consecutive ablation sessions in the era of computer assisted image guidance—Lessons learned. European Journal of Radiology. 2019;**6**:1-8. Available from: http://www.ncbi.nlm.nih.gov/pubmed/30547062

[35] Fuhrmann I, Probst U, Wiggermann P, Beyer L. Navigation systems for treatment planning and execution of percutaneous irreversible electroporation. Technology in Cancer Research & Treatment. 2018;**17**:153303381879179. Available from: http://www.ncbi.nlm.nih.gov/pubmed/30071779

[36] Martin RCG, North DA. Enhanced ultrasound with navigation leads to improved liver lesion identification and needle placement. The Journal of Surgical Research. 2016;**200**(2):420-426. Available from: https://www.sciencedirect.com/science/article/pii/S0022480415008847?via%3Dihub

[37] Lachenmayer A, Tinguely P, Maurer MH, Frehner L, Knöpfli M, Peterhans M, et al. Stereotactic image-guided microwave ablation of hepatocellular carcinoma using a computer-assisted navigation system. Liver International. 2019;**39**(10):1975-1985. DOI: 10.1111/liv.14187

[38] Beyer LP, Pregler B, Michalik K, Niessen C, Dollinger M, Müller M, et al. Evaluation of a robotic system for irreversible electroporation (IRE) of malignant liver tumors: Initial results. International Journal of Computer Assisted Radiology and Surgery. 2017;**12**(5):803-809

[39] Beyer LP, Pregler B, Nießen C, Schicho A, Haimerl M, Jung EM, et al. Stereotactically-navigated percutaneous Irreversible Electroporation (IRE) compared to conventional IRE: a prospective trial. PeerJ. 2016;**4**(8):e2277. Available from: http://www.ncbi.nlm.nih.gov/pubmed/27602266

[40] Teatini A, Pelanis E, Aghayan DL, Kumar RP, Palomar R, Fretland ÅA, et al. The effect of intraoperative

imaging on surgical navigation for laparoscopic liver resection surgery. Scientific Reports. 2019;**9**(1):18687. Available from: http://www.nature.com/articles/s41598-019-54915-3

[41] Prevost GA, Eigl B, Paolucci I, Rudolph T, Peterhans M, Weber S, et al. Efficiency, accuracy and clinical applicability of a new image-guided surgery system in 3D laparoscopic liver surgery. Journal of Gastrointestinal Surgery. 2019;**16**:1-8

[42] Stillström D, Nilsson H, Jesse M, Peterhans M, Jonas E, Freedman J. A new technique for minimally invasive irreversible electroporation of tumors in the head and body of the pancreas. Surgical Endoscopy. 2016;**31**(4):1-4. Available from: http://www.ncbi.nlm.nih.gov/pubmed/27572065

[43] Wallach D, Toporek G, Weber S, Bale R, Widmann G. Comparison of freehand-navigated and aiming device-navigated targeting of liver lesions. International Journal of Medical Robotics and Computer Assisted Surgery. 2014;**10**(1):35-43

[44] Durand P, Moreau-Gaudry A, Silvent AS, Frandon J, Chipon E, Médici M, et al. Computer assisted electromagnetic navigation improves accuracy in computed tomography guided interventions: A prospective randomized clinical trial. PLoS One. 2017;**12**(3)

[45] Bond L, Schulz B, VanMeter T, Martin RCG. Intra-operative navigation of a 3-dimensional needle localization system for precision of irreversible electroporation needles in locally advanced pancreatic cancer. European Journal of Surgical Oncology. 2017;**43**(2):337-343. Available from: https://www.sciencedirect.com/science/article/pii/S0748798316308988?via%3Dihub

[46] Ben-David E, Ahmed M, Faroja M, Moussa M, Wandel A, Sosna J, et al. Irreversible electroporation: Treatment effect is susceptible to local environment and tissue properties. Radiology. 2013;**269**(3):738-747

[47] He XF, Xiao YY, Zhang X, Zhang XB, Zhang X, Wei YT, et al. Preliminary clinical application of the robot-assisted CT-guided irreversible electroporation ablation for the treatment of pancreatic head carcinoma. International Journal of Medical Robotics and Computer Assisted Surgery. 2020;**16**(4). Available from: https://onlinelibrary.wiley.com/doi/abs/10.1002/rcs.2099

[48] Rashid MF, Hecht EM, Steinman JA, Kluger MD. Irreversible electroporation of pancreatic adenocarcinoma: A primer for the radiologist. Abdominal Radiology (New York). 2018;**43**(2):457-466

[49] Litjens G, Kooi T, Bejnordi BE, Setio AAA, Ciompi F, Ghafoorian M, et al. A survey on deep learning in medical image analysis. Medical Image Analysis. 2017;**42**:60-88

[50] Bagheri MH, Roth H, Kovacs W, Yao J, Farhadi F, Li X, et al. Technical and clinical factors affecting success rate of a deep learning method for pancreas segmentation on CT. Academic Radiology. 2019

[51] Roth HR, Shen C, Oda H, Sugino T, Oda M, Hayashi Y, et al. A multi-scale pyramid of 3D fully convolutional networks for abdominal multi-organ segmentation. In: Lecture Notes in Computer Science (including subseries Lecture Notes in Artificial Intelligence and Lecture Notes in Bioinformatics). Springer Verlag; 2018. pp. 417-425. DOI: 10.1007/978-3-030-00937-3_48

[52] Baegert C, Villard C, Schreck P, Soler L, Gangi A. Trajectory optimization for the planning of percutaneous radiofrequency ablation of hepatic tumors. Computer Aided Surgery. 2007;**12**(2):82-90

[53] Au JT, Kingham TP, Jun K, Haddad D, Gholami S, Mojica K, et al. Irreversible electroporation ablation of the liver can be detected with ultrasound B-mode and elastography. Surgery. 2013;**153**(6):787-793. Available from: https://linkinghub.elsevier.com/retrieve/pii/S0039606012007350

[54] Bhutiani N, Doughtie CA, Martin RCG. Ultrasound validation of mathematically modeled irreversible electroporation ablation areas. Surgery. 2016;**159**(4):1032-1040. Available from: http://linkinghub.elsevier.com/retrieve/pii/S0039606015009071

Chapter 5

Current Systemic Treatment Options for Metastatic and Unresectable Pancreatic Cancer

Christian Caglevic, Mauricio Mahave,
Cristobal Sanhueza and Luis Ubillos

Abstract

Metastatic and local advanced unresectable pancreatic cancers are lethal conditions that always carry a poor prognosis with rare exceptions. Currently, the mainstay of therapy is cytotoxic chemotherapy plus best supportive care. First-line therapy for patients with a good performance status includes FOLFIRINOX or gemcitabine plus nab-paclitaxel regimens. Patients carrying a deleterious germline BRCA mutation can be treated with maintenance olaparib after FOLFIRINOX. Patients with a poor performance status, but still fit enough for chemotherapy, may be treated with single agent gemcitabine. Second-line therapy will depend on previous therapy and current performance status. Options for patients treated with gemcitabine-based regimens are 5-fluorouracil plus leucovorin plus either nanoliposomal irinotecan, irinotecan or oxaliplatin. Patients that were treated with first line FOLFIRINOX may benefit from a gemcitabine-based chemotherapy, but evidence from randomized trials is lacking. Other options like immunotherapy and targeted therapies yield benefit only in very selected cases, and it is still an area of research.

Keywords: metastatic pancreatic cancer, unresectable pancreatic cancer, local advanced pancreatic cancer, FOLFIRINOX, nab-paclitaxel, gemcitabine, nanoliposomal irinotecan, olaparib, BRCA pancreatic cancer

1. Introduction

Advanced exocrine pancreatic cancer (PC) is one of the most lethal malignancies among all types of solid tumors. According to data from United States of America (USA) registries, 29% of the patients will debut with locally advanced disease, and 53% will have metastases at diagnosis [1]. Even in the cases when resection is feasible, long-term survival rates are among 3.9 and 9.3%, meanwhile 5 years-overall survival for stage IV is lesser than 3% [1, 2]. The late stage at presentation and the particular microenvironment characterized by predominant desmoplastic tissue and immunosuppressive cells explain why PC poses such a challenge [3].

Historically, median overall survival (mOS) for advanced stages was around 6 months when the patient was treated with gemcitabine or gemcitabine-based

IntechOpen

combinations but new chemotherapy regimens and better understanding of the tumor biology has led to improved, yet still poor, survival [4].

Unlike other cancers, target therapy has yielded only modest benefit in PC. There are only two targeted agents than historically have got approval for metastatic or unresectable PC: erlotinib and olaparib. Erlotinib, a tyrosine kinase inhibitor (TKi) targeting the epidermal grow factor receptor (EGFR), in combination with gemcitabine, when compared with gemcitabine alone, showed a statistically significant, but clinically modest benefit in OS [5]. Just recently, the US Food and Drug Administration (FDA) approved the PARP inhibitor olaparib for PC in patients with deleterious or suspected deleterious germline BRCA mutations [6], which are present only in approximately 5% of pancreatic cancer patients.

Immunotherapy has showed great advances in melanoma and lung cancer among others, has not yield any promising results in PC. The site agnostic FDA approval for checkpoint inhibitors for mismatch repair deficient tumors (dMMR) or tumors with high microsatellite instability (MSI-H) has modest impact in PC [7], given that those abnormalities are infrequent in pancreatic adenocarcinoma.

Current research is looking for development of new drugs with different mechanisms of action in order to overcome chemotherapy resistance wishing to improve survival and quality of life in advanced PC patients.

Considering that pancreatic cancer is mainly a systemic disease we have focused this chapter in systemic treatments addressed to unrecoverable patients and we will not refer here to local treatments such as radiation therapy or chemoradiation that can be curative in a very small amount of patients but that do not have a real impact in survival in the metastatic or micrometastatic scenario.

2. First steps: chemotherapy development in metastatic or unresectable pancreatic adenocarcinoma

Earlier tested in gastric cancer by the Southwest Oncology Group the combination of 5-Fluoruracil, Adriamycin and Mitomycin C (FAM) was later assessed in advanced PC patients and published in 1980. Smith et al. reported a 37% of partial responses (PR) and 11% of stable disease (SD) among 27 patients that were treated with this regimen and had measurable disease, with a median duration of response (mDOR) of 9 months. Patients with better performance status were more likely to response (55%) and patients with Performance Status (PS)2–3 only achieved a 29% of response rate (RR) ($p < 0.15$). Median OS was higher in patients that responded (12 months) when compared with nonresponders (3.5 months) ($p < 0.01$). Myelosuppression was the most relevant toxicity reported in this trial [8].

In 1985, a multicenter phase 3 clinical trial that compared 5-Fluoruracil (5FU) alone or in combination with Adriamycin (FA) or in combination with Adriamycin plus Mitomycin C (FAM) in treating advanced pancreatic and gastric carcinoma was published. This trial that included 144 PC patients from 11 centers of the United States with advanced or metastatic adenocarcinoma of the pancreas, did not show any benefit of both combination arms when compared with 5-FU alone in terms of median OS, median time to progression (TTP), objective response rate (ORR) and parameters of palliation, however, the reported hematological and nonhematological toxicities were higher in the FA and FAM arms when compared with 5 FU alone [9]. This clinical trial led to a decreasing use of FAM regimen and for the increasing need to look for new treatments for these population of patients.

3. Gemcitabine: a new era for pancreatic cancer

One decade later, gemcitabine, a nucleoside analogue that exhibits antitumor activity, started to show promising results in PC patients.

Conducted as a phase 2 trial by former concepts, Casper et al. reported their experience of treating 44 PC patients, all of them with confirmed adenocarcinoma, not amenable to curative surgical treatment, performance status 0–1, and measurable disease (32 patients with metastatic disease and 12 patients with local advanced PC). The initial dose of gemcitabine was 800 mg/m^2 weekly for 3 weeks and 1 week off. Thirty-five patients received two or more cycles of Gemcitabine. Median TTP was 16 weeks. Five patients (11%) achieved a major response according to the radiological criteria used in the trial, the median duration of response for those patients was 13 months but only 5.6 months for all the treated population. Reported one-year survival was 23%. Most of the patients presented mild toxicity to gemcitabine including hematological, cutaneous toxicity, alopecia, nausea, vomiting and diarrhea. Some of these patients were treated with increasing doses of Gemcitabine, 1000 mg/m^2 then 1250 mg/m^2 and 2 patients up to 1500 mg/m^2; however, those last patients needed a reduction of their doses due to flu-like syndrome [4].

In a phase 3 randomized clinical trial Gemcitabine was compared head to head with 5 FU. This study included 126 patients from Canada and the United States with locally-advanced-unresectable or metastatic PC. Despite the known limited benefit of 5-FU in PC the investigators that designed the trial decided to use it as control arm instead of a placebo arm. The primary end point for this trial was "Clinical Benefit" (considering analgesic consumption, pain intensity, performance status and weight); secondary end points included response rate, time to disease progression and survival. Gemcitabine was given as a 1000 mg/m^2 intravenous regimen weekly for 7 weeks and 1 week of rest, followed by 1000 mg/m^2 weekly during 3 weeks with 1 week of rest during the rest of the treatment. 5-FU was given weekly in a fixed dose of 600 mg/m^2 intravenously. Primary end point was met, and this resulted in a positive trial achieving a clinical benefit of 23.8% in the gemcitabine arm and only 4.8% in the 5 FU arm. Median OS and TTP were 5.6 months and 9 weeks for gemcitabine arm versus 4.4 months and 4 weeks for 5FU arm, reported 12-months survival was 18 and 2% for gemcitabine and 5FU respectively ($p = 0.0025$). Among gemcitabine treated patients only a 5.4% achieved a radiological response but none from the 5 FU arm did, 39 and 19% of SD was reported for both arms. When compared responders versus nonresponder median OS was 10.7 months versus 4.8 months regardless of the treatment arm. Grade 3–4 neutropenia was higher in the gemcitabine arm (25.9% versus 4.9% for 5-FU, $p < 0.001$), No severe infections were reported in either arms but grade 3 and 4 anemia was 9.7% in gemcitabine arm and 0% in 5 FU arm, grade 1–2 fever was higher in gemcitabine arm 30.1% versus 16% for 5-FU, rashes 23.8 versus 12.9%, grade 3–4 nausea vomiting 9.5 and 3.2% versus 4.8 and 0% respectively. For both arms there were no survivors after 19 months since starting treatment [10]. This trial led to FDA to approve Gemcitabine as a first line of treatment for unresectable or metastatic pancreatic cancer in 1996.

Due to the positive results of gemcitabine in patients with advanced PC many combinations of gemcitabine-based treatments were tested looking to improve OS and progression free survival (PFS), most of them did not show improvement in overall survival as shown in HU's meta-analysis [11]: gemcitabine—5-FU combination (conducted by J. D. Berlin); gemcitabine—irinotecan combination (trials conducted by G. Rocha Lima and by G.P. Stathopoulos); gemcitabine—oxaliplatin (trials conducted by C. Louvet and by E. Poplin); gemcitabine—pemetrexed (conducted by H Oettle); gemcitabine—exatecan (conducted by G. Abou-Alfa); gemcitabine—cisplatin (trials conducted by V. Heinemann and by G. Colucci); gemcitabine—capecitabine (conducted by D. Cunningham); gemcitabine—bevacizumab (conducted by H. Kindler); gemcitabine—cetuximab (conducted by P. Philip); gemcitabine—axitinib (conducted by H. Kindler). Gemcitabine—sorafenib combination also resulted in negative trials in terms of overall survival [12].

Despite those several negative clinical trials, a meta-analysis conducted by Ciliberto aimed to evaluate the role of gemcitabine-based combination therapy when compared with gemcitabine alone. Including more than 10.600 patients from 34 randomized trials, the combination treatments showed marginal superiority in terms of survival, overall response, and disease control rate but with higher toxicity rates mainly diarrhea, nausea, neutropenia, thrombocytopenia. One of the interpretations of the authors was that combination regimens gemcitabine-based should be reserved only for well selected patient populations [13]. In an Asiatic population study, a 3-arms clinical trial was conducted to compare gemcitabine alone, gemcitabine plus S-1 combination or S-1 alone in local advanced and in metastatic pancreatic patients. The combination arm did not show superiority when compared with gemcitabine alone, however, S-1 showed noninferiority against gemcitabine with a good tolerability profile [14].

From PC biopsies Fjallskog et al. found and reported that 55% of tumor samples studied stained positive for Epidermal Growth Factor Receptor (EGFR) [15]. In a murine model of pancreatic adenocarcinoma adding erlotinib highly inhibited gemcitabine-induced MAP kinase signaling regardless of the activation of KRAS by maintaining high levels of ERBB2 protein [16]. A multicenter phase 3 double blind international trial assessed gemcitabine plus erlotinib combination versus gemcitabine plus placebo [5]. About 569 patients with unresectable or metastatic adenocarcinoma of the pancreas, ECOG 0–2 were randomized in a 1:1 ratio to receive either gemcitabine alone or gemcitabine plus erlotinib. Gemcitabine was given intravenously 1000 mg/m^2 weekly for 7 weeks and 1 week off, then 1000 mg/m^2 weekly for 3 weeks and 1 week off during the next cycles (28 days cycle). Erlotinib was orally given in a 100 mg dose and increased to 150 mg in a Canadian cohort. The primary end point was OS, secondary end points included PFS, ORR, duration of response, correlation of EGFR expression with outcomes, quality of life and toxicity. Reported median survival and one-year survival were 6.24 months and 23% for the gemcitabine—erlotinib arm versus 5.9 months and 17% for the gemcitabine-placebo arm. PFS was improved in the combination arm. Despite these positive results in statistical terms, the clinical value was marginal and the reported toxicity significantly higher in the combination arm, including 6 deaths protocol-related all of them in patients in the gemcitabine-erlotinib arm including interstitial pneumonitis, sepsis, stroke and neutropenic sepsis. Immunohistochemical analysis and correlation with response did not show any improvement among EGFR positive patients. Interestingly, patients that developed skin rash grade 2 or higher lived longer when compared with whom did not (10.5 months for grade 2 versus 5.8 months and 5.3 months for grade 1 and 0 respectively), 1-year survival was 16% for rash grade, 0, 9% for rash grade 1 and 43% for rash grade 2 or higher ($p < 0.001$).

A German trial that compared erlotinib in combination with either capecitabine or gemcitabine as the front-line treatment for advanced pancreatic cancer patients allowing cross over after failure showed a low toxicity rate for both arms and not deaths treatment-related [17].

Despite that gemcitabine-erlotinib combination got FDA approval for metastatic or unresectable PC, considering its minimal benefit in terms of survival when compared with gemcitabine alone and also due to the higher toxicity profile of the combination, it is not considered as a "first option of treatment" in advanced pancreatic adenocarcinoma patient by different authors and international guidelines [18, 19].

4. 2020: current first-line options for the treatment of metastatic and or unresectable adenocarcinoma of the pancreas and their historical development

Based on the knowledge from preclinical assays and clinical studies that had showed synergist activity of irinotecan, oxaliplatin and 5-FU combination, a phase 1 trial assessed a regimen that combined 5-FU, leucovorin. Irinotecan and oxaliplatin [20]. This trial included 34 patients with different malignancies, 6 of them with pancreatic advanced cancer. Among pancreatic cancer patients one partial response and one complete response were achieved. For all the patients treated main grade 3–4 toxicities included 78% neutropenia (12% febrile neutropenia), 41% asthenia, 37% peripheral neuropathy, 27% diarrhea and 24% nausea and vomiting, 6% thrombocytopenia and 5% anemia. 51% of the patients required granulocyte colony stimulating factor (G-CSF).

FOLFIRINOX regimen (oxaliplatin 85 mg/m^2 + Irinotecan 180 mg/m^2 + Leucovorin 400 mg/m^2 + 5-FU 400 mg/m^2 in bolus and 5-FU 2400 mg/m^2 in 46 hours in continuous infusion) every 2 weeks was evaluated in a phase 2 French clinical trial that included 46 patients with advanced or metastatic pancreatic adenocarcinoma that had not received previous treatment (chemotherapy, radiotherapy or chemoradiation), with ages between 18 and 70 years, performance status 0–1, adequate bone marrow function, total bilirubin not superior than 1.5 times the upper normal level (UNL), AST – ALT and alkaline phosphatases <3 ULN (5 < ULN in patients with liver metastasis) and an adequate renal function were some of the selection criteria [21]. Patients with brain or leptomeningeal disease were excluded. Primary end point of the trial was response rate end according to former WHO criteria; secondary end points included safety, quality of life and clinical benefit assessment. Treatment was given until progression of disease or unacceptable toxicity for up to 6 months of chemotherapy in case of benefit. According to protocol atropine was allowed to be administered to diminish the risk of severe cholinergic syndrome in patients that presented it in a previous cycle. Antiemetic prophylaxis treatment was permitted at investigator's discretion. Loperamide was allowed for patients with delayed diarrhea and oral fluroquinolones in case that diarrhea lasted more than 2 days. After cycle 1 of treatment G-CSFs were also allowed to be used in case of need. The median of age of patients was 56 years, 65% were male and 76% stage IV B, doses reductions were indicated in the 14% of the total of cycles for all the patients. Most of delays for new cycles were due to hematological toxicities. By investigators assessment and after a median follow up of 33 months, the overall response rate was 26% (all partial responses) and 39% of patients achieved stable disease, the median duration of response was 10.4 months, PFS was 5.6 months, median OS was 10.2 months (9.5 months for metastatic patients and 15.7 months for locally advanced disease), 1-year survival was 43%. Grade 3–4 neutropenia occurred in the 52% of patients but only 4% of febrile neutropenia was reported, 8% of treated patients need hospitalization due to diarrhea, grade 3 and 4 vomiting was 20 and 17%, grade 3 and 4 asthenia was 20 and 21%, grade 2 and 3 peripheral neuropathy was 13 and 15% respectively and 7 patients were discontinued of treatment for this last toxicity. Concerning quality of life 18% of patients reported worsening and 37% reported improvement in quality of life.

By those days, the standard of care for advanced PC gemcitabine was compared head to head against FOLFIRINOX regimen in a first line of treatment, multicenter phase 2–3 clinical trial designed by the same French group [22]. About 342 patients were randomized in a 1:1 ratio to receive either FOLFIRINOX every 2 weeks at the same doses than in the phase 2 trial or gemcitabine that was given intravenously 1000 mg/m^2 weekly during 7 weeks and 1 week off, then 1000 mg/m^2 weekly during 3 weeks and 1 week of rest. Main inclusion criteria were age 18 years or older, histologically or cytologically confirmed adenocarcinoma of the pancreas, measurable disease, ECOG 0–1 and adequate hepatic, renal and bone marrow function. Exclusion criteria included but were not limited to an age older than 76 years, previous radiotherapy for measurable lesions, brain metastases and others.

OS was the primary end point of this trial. Secondary end points included PFS, tumor response, safety and quality of life. The median number of cycles was 10 for FOLFIRINOX arm (range 1–47) and 6 for Gemcitabine (range 1–26) ($p < 0.001$). With a median follow up of 26 months median OS was 11.1 months for FOLFIRINOX arm and 6.8 months for Gemcitabine arm (HR 0.57; $p < 0.001$). Reported survival rates at 6–12-18 months were 57.6–20.6% and 6% for gemcitabine arm and 75.9, 48.4, 18.6% for FOLFIRINOX arm. According to RECIST criteria there was a 31.6% of responses among the FOLFIRINOX treated patients including 1 complete response but also 38.6% of stable disease as the best response. For the gemcitabine arm it was reported a 41.5% of stable disease and only a 9.4% of partial responses. Median PFS was 6.4 months and 3.3 months for FOLFIRINOX and Gemcitabine arms respectively (HR 0.47; $p < 0.001$). Patients that received a second line of therapy had a median OS de 4.4 months in each group since new treatment started. Grade 3 and 4 toxicities were more frequent in the FOLFIRINOX arm including neutropenia, febrile neutropenia, thrombocytopenia, diarrhea, peripheral neuropathy and also grade 2 alopecia. ALT elevations were significatively higher among gemcitabine treated patients. 42% of the FOLFIRINOX-treated patients required G-CSF but only 5% of the patients of the gemcitabine arm. At a 6 months period 66% of gemcitabine treated patients and 31% in the FOLFIRINOX arm had a decrease in the scores of quality of life (HR 0.47; $p < 0.01$). Later reports from the same group remarked about the risk of worsening in quality of life among patients treated with FOLFIRINOX regimen when compared with gemcitabine-treated patients [23].

Based on the results of this French trial, FOLFIRINOX has shown to be superior in terms of OS, PFS and ORR, and it is currently worldwide accepted as a first line option of treatment for patients with advanced PC, however, it is necessary to remember that this regimen was approved in patients younger of 76 years old and it was assessed only in French population.

Some authors have reported their experiences in patients using some modifications of the FOLFIRINOX regimen (known as modified FOLFIRINOX or mFOLFIRINOX). Considering a significant dispersion of results among them, some retrospective analysis and meta- analysis showed similar results in terms of survival but with less toxicity when compared with the results from the pivotal study mentioned above [24]. Avoiding 5-FU bolus and using hematopoietic growth factors also seems to be safe in mFOLFIRINOX regimen when it is used in metastatic pancreatic cancer [25].

Before FOLFIRINOX was recognized as the first option of treatment for advanced disease the standard of treatment was gemcitabine. Gemcitabine has lower efficacy but a better toxicity profile when compared with FOLFIRINOX and it can still be used in the first line of treatment among patients that are not amenable to receive FOLFIRINOX or gemcitabine-nab paclitaxel combination. Nab-paclitaxel is a derivate, solvent-free, albumin bound form of paclitaxel with some relevant advantages over paclitaxel including a significant lower hypersensitivity reactions profile and a shorter infusion time. Its formulation with albumin also allows nab-paclitaxel to reach the tumor microenvironment by using endogenous albumin transport pathways [26]. A glycoprotein that has been related in the carcinogenesis of several solid tumors, SPARC (secreted protein acidic and rich in cysteine), has been found in high levels in the tumor stroma of pancreatic cancer, mainly in peritumoral fibroblasts and it has been linked with bad prognosis. In complete resected patients 5-year survival has been reported to be worse among pancreatic cancer patients that express stromal SPARC and it might be considered as a prognostic marker [27]. Tumor stroma's SPARC seems to facilitate that nab-paclitaxel penetrates the tumor microenvironment hypothesizing that this drug may have a significant potential role in the pancreatic cancer control [28].

As earlier mentioned in this chapter, gemcitabine was combined with several other drugs looking to improve survival and quality of life in advanced PC, unfortunately those trials` outcomes were mostly negative. One exception was gemcitabine plus Nab-paclitaxel combination that is currently another recommended first-line treatment option in the metastatic setting of patients harboring adenocarcinoma of the pancreas. Comparing nab-paclitaxel with other chemotherapy agents, there is evidence of synergism in a mouse model when gemcitabine was combined with nab-paclitaxel by reducing cytidine deaminase levels that involves gemcitabine's metabolism [29].

A phase 1–2 clinical trial was conducted to define the maximum tolerated dose (MTD) of gemcitabine plus Nab-paclitaxel combination in previously untreated metastatic PC patients. The regimen was then finally defined as gemcitabine 1000 mg/m^2 plus nab paclitaxel 125 mg/m^2 weekly for 3 weeks every 28 days. Reported dose limiting toxicities were mainly neutropenia and sepsis. Outcomes from patients treated with the MTD showed a 1-year survival of 48%, with a median OS of 12.2 months and a response rate of 48%. Interestingly, as part of this trial FDG PET CT response was also assessed and showed that patients with complete metabolic response had a longer overall survival of 20.1 months versus 10.3 months in patients that did not achieve a metabolic complete response ($p = 0.01$) [30].

Von Hoff et al., following the previous phase 1–2 trial, designed an international multicenter open label phase 3 clinical trial to compare gemcitabine plus nab-paclitaxel combination with gemcitabine alone in patients with advanced PC (MPACT trial) [31]. The study arm used the same doses of gemcitabine and nab-paclitaxel suggested by the previous phase1–2 trial. The control arm, gemcitabine alone was given in a dose of 1000 mg/m^2 weekly for 7 weeks in an 8 weeks cycle (defines as protocol as cycle 1) and then 1000 mg/m^2 weekly for 3 weeks every 4 weeks. The primary end point was OS and secondary end points included PFS and ORR. Inclusion criteria included patients with a confirmed metastatic adenocarcinoma of the pancreas with measurable disease by RECIST 1.0, Karnofsky score of 70–100, chemotherapy naive (patients that received previous gemcitabine or 5-FU as radiosensitizers were allowed to participate in the trial), adequate renal, bone marrow and liver function as defined by protocol. Patients that had received adjuvant chemotherapy and patients with locally advance disease were excluded. Stratification was according to Karfnofsky score, presence or not of liver metastases and geographical region. Randomization was performed in a 1:1 ratio and the trial included 861 patients (63% from North America, 15% from Eastern Europe, 14% from Australia and 9% from western Europe). 10% of patients were older than 75 years and 8% of patients had ECOG 2. The primary end point of the trial was met, median OS was 8.5 months for the combination arm and 6>7 months for the gemcitabine alone group (HR 0.72; $p < 0.001$). 1 and 2-year survival were higher for the gemcitabine plus nab-paclitaxel combination arm (35 and 9%) arm when compared with gemcitabine alone (9 and 4%). Patients that underwent a second line of treatment lived longer if they had been treated with the combination treatment (9.4 months for gemcitabine-nab paclitaxel versus 6.8 months for gemcitabine alone, HR 0.68; $p < 0.001$). PFS, ORR and disease control rate (DCR) were also higher in the combination arm: PFS 5.5 months versus 3.7 months

(HR 0.69, $p < 0.001$), ORR 23% versus 7% ($p < 0.001$) and DCR of-16 weeks-or-longer 48% versus 33% respectively ($p < 0.001$). In addition, patients that had a decrease in basal CA 19–9 of 90% or more irrespective of the treatment arm live longer when compared with patients that reached a decrease of this biomarker lower than 90% (13.5 months versus 8.2 months, HR 0.53; $p < 0.001$). 15% of patients from gemcitabine arm and 32% of the combination arm received at least 6 months of treatment. Reported grade 3–4 toxicities were higher among gemcitabine-nab paclitaxel arm (neutropenia 38 vs. 27%, leukopenia 31 vs. 16%, fatigue 17 vs. 7%, peripheral neuropathy 17 vs. 1%, diarrhea 6 vs. 1%). Discontinuation of nab paclitaxel due to peripheral neuropathy grade 1–3 was 8% and no grade 4 neuropathy was reported. 3% of patients in the combination arm developed febrile neutropenia and 26% receipted G-CSF versus 1 and 15% for gemcitabine arm respectively. There was a 4% of fatal events in each group but sepsis and pneumonitis related deaths were more frequent among gemcitabine plus nab paclitaxel treated patients.

Un update of the long-term survival of this trial was later published [32]. The median OS for the gemcitabine-nab paclitaxel combination was 8.7 months versus 6.6 months for the gemcitabine arm (HR 0.72; $p < 0.001$). Patients that lived 3 years or longer was only a 4% and they all had been treated with the combination treatment. Higher CA 19–9 and neutrophil to lymphocyte ratio > 5 were associated with worse survival and there was a trend for more benefit in those poor prognosis subgroups.

The phase 2 multicenter, international, single arm LAPACT trial was addressed to assess the efficacy and safety of gemcitabine plus Nab-paclitaxel combination in patients with locally advanced, unresectable nonmetastatic, previously untreated pancreatic cancer [33]. Primary end point was time to treatment failure (TTF). This study was designed for all the patients to be treated in a "induction phase" with gemcitabine 1000 mg/m^2 plus nab-paclitaxel 125 mg/m^2 weekly for 3 weeks in a 28 days cycle for a total of 6 cycles. After this induction period, patients without disease progression, by investigator choice, were treated with the same chemotherapy regimen or chemoradiation or surgery (patients with responses before this 6 cycles period could undergo surgery without have to end the complete all pre-programmed chemotherapy treatment). Only ECOG 0–1 patients were allowed to be enrolled. A total of 106 patients were evaluable. Median TTF was 8.6 months and PFS 10.2 months. Main reasons for discontinuing treatment were adverse events (18%) and progressive disease (7%). Grade 3 or higher toxicity reported included 42% neutropenia, 11% anemia, 10% fatigue and 4% of peripheral neuropathy. Respecting to efficacy to treatment 32.7% of patients had a partial response and 57.9% stable disease as the best reported response. 43% of patients continue treatment with gemcitabine plus nab paclitaxel after induction treatment, 16% underwent chemoradiation and 15% of patients underwent surgery (n 16). Of the 16 patients that underwent surgery, 7 patients achieved a R0 resection and 9 patients a R1 resection.

This chemotherapy regimen, gemcitabine plus nab-paclitaxel combination, is currently also an option to consider for unresectable patients, with a very low curative option, in tumors that have a real minor chance to undergo a R0 resection, as it has already been already described for FOLFIRINOX and chemoradiation [34, 35].

No phase 3 clinical trial has compared the efficacy of FOLFIRINOX and gemcitabine plus nab-paclitaxel combination, for this reason selection of patients for either treatment must consider the differences between both phase 3 pivotal trials. The phase 2 trial LAPACT also provide us some information for unresectable patients that underwent gemcitabine- nab paclitaxel treatment looking for a neoadjuvant option considering that phase 3 trial MPACT only enrolled metastatic patients. MPACT trial allowed the inclusion of patients older than 75 years (10%)

and poorer performance status (8% ECOG 2), in the FOLFIRINOX phase 3 trial patients older than 75 years were not allowed and ECOG was limited to <2. Despite that FOLFIRINOX trial was a multicenter only included French sites, however, MPACT included patients from North America, Europe, and Australia.

A systematic meta-analysis aimed to answer if there is superiority of FOLFIRINOX or gemcitabine-nab paclitaxel combination in the first line of treatment for metastatic or advanced PC. Based on 16 retrospective studies that included 2123 gemcitabine plus nab-paclitaxel treated patients and 1690 FOLFIRINOX treated patients, no statistical significantly differences were found in terms of overall risk of death, PFS and RR. Toxicity was in line of the pivotal trials [36]. These results may help to conclude that despite of the numerically superiority in OS of the phase 3 FOLFIRINOX trial when it is compared with MPACT trial, and in the absence of a comparative head to head phase 3 trial for these 2 regimens, clinicians may use any of those according with their experience but also taking account of the medical conditions and biography of each patient to be treated.

BRCA 1–2 mutations have been found between the 5% and 12.8% of pancreatic cancer patients among different patient populations [6]. In a retrospective observational study that analyzed the outcomes in 71 PC patients harboring BRCA 1–2 germline mutations, OS was statistically higher among stage 3–4 patients that were treated with platinum-based chemotherapy when compared with patients that did not use platin compounds as part of their treatment (22 versus 9 months, $p = 0.039$) [37].

Recently published, the POLO study (Pancreas Cancer Olaparib Ongoing) was a phase 3 multicenter doble blinded in patients with metastatic PC and BRCA1–2 germline mutations that had received at least 16 weeks of a platinum-based palliative chemotherapy and had no disease progression during the treatment, then patients were assigned to receive olaparib (300 mg twice daily) or placebo in a 2:1 ratio [38]. The primary end point of the trial was PFS by a blinded independent central review. 154 patients were randomized (3315 patients screened). 86% of the olaparib group and 81% of the placebo group had been treated with FOLFIRINOX regimen and 2 and 5% with gemcitabine cisplatin combination, respectively. Primary end point, PFS was met showing longer median PFS among patients treated with olaparib versus placebo (7.4 versus 3.8 months, HR 0.53, $p = 0.004$), however, no benefit in overall survival was found for 18.9 months in olaparib arm and 18.1 months in placebo arm ($p = 0.68$). 23% of patients olaparib-treated had response (including 2 patients that achieved a complete response) vs. 12% in the placebo arm by blinded independent central review, with a median duration of response of 24.9 versus 3.7 months respectively. Considering that POLO trial resulted in a positive trial achieving to meet its primary end point PFS, FDA in December 2019 got the approval for the use of olaparib for the maintenance treatment of adult patients with germline BRCA-mutated metastatic adenocarcinoma of the pancreas without disease progression on at least 16 weeks of a first-line platinum-based chemotherapy regimen such as FOLFIRINOX and cisplatin-based chemotherapy. This way, olaparib became the first drug to be approved as a maintenance treatment for pancreatic cancer and currently is a new weapon to improve PFS among BRCA-mutated PC patients.

5. Second-line systemic therapy for metastatic or local advanced unresectable adenocarcinoma of the pancreas

After progression to a first-line therapy, subsequent treatment will depend greatly on the patient performance status and which drugs were or not given before.

Other factors to take in account are molecular abnormalities like dMMR/MSI-H or mutations that can be targeted (druggable mutations).

Patient that received gemcitabine-based chemotherapy as the first-line therapy can be treated with a combination of 5-FU and nanoliposomal irinotecan (nal-IRI). The phase III Napoli-1 trial showed an overall survival difference of 1.9 months (6.1 versus 4.2) when compared with 5-fluorouracil monotherapy (HR 0.67) [39]. 45% of the patients had received 5-FU treatment as a previous line, but only 10% of the patients had received irinotecan previously. A subgroup analysis showed that the benefit was maintained in patients that had received 5-FU but not in those previously treated with irinotecan. A recent update of this trial showed an estimated 1-year survival of 26% for nanoliposomal irinotecan plus 5-FU combination versus 16% for 5 FU alone [40].

Nanoliposomal irinotecan is not yet widely available. Phase two trials have shown than irinotecan plus 5-fluorouracil and leucovorin (FOLFIRI) has modest activity, but comparable to nal-Iri, in patients previously treated with gemcitabine, with an overall response rate of 15% and 35% of stable disease, time to progression 3.7 months and median OS of 6 months [41, 42]. The 2018 American Society of Clinical Oncology (ASCO) guidelines for treatment of metastatic PC endorses the use of FOLFIRI in countries were nal-Iri is not available [43].

Oxaliplatin-containing regimens such as FOLFOX or oxaliplatin plus 5-FU have yielded mixed results as a second line in this setting, with poor accrual and modest benefit. The multicenter German phase III Conko-003 trial compared OFF regimen (oxaliplatin, folinic acid and fluorouracil) against fluorouracil and folinic acid (FF) in patients that had disease progression after gemcitabine treatment. This trial resulted positive in terms of overall survival (median overall survival 5.9 months for OFF regimen and 3.3 months for FF regimen, HR 0.66 $p = 0.01$) and in terms of time to progression (2.9 months for OFF and 2.0 months for FF respectively, HR 0.68, $p = 0.19$). Reported neurotoxicity grade 1–2 was higher among OFF- treated patients (38% versus 7% in FF group) [44]. Conversely, the phase III PANCREOX trial failed to show benefit for FOLFOX as second line therapy as compared to 5FU single therapy [45]. With those results, oxaliplatin based regimens are less preferred than nal-Iri or irinotecan-based regimens, but still an option in patients who cannot receive the latter for any circumstances and are still fit and willing to pursue further therapy.

When the combination of irinotecan, oxaliplatin, leucovorin and 5FU (FOLFIRINOX) regimen is given as a first line therapy, patient in good shape could be treated with a gemcitabine-based regimen. Reports have shown feasibility of this regimen [46, 47], but there are no phase III trials supporting this recommendation. As a result, from first line chemotherapy toxicity and declined performance status, it is advisable to use an attenuated regimen in this situation, reducing doses or changing schedules to biweekly administration [48].

Patients with poor performance status, but still fit enough and willing to receive further therapy, should not receive multiagent regimens. Gemcitabine or 5-FU single drug could represent an option for those patients, given the toxicities associated with more intense regimens and modest benefit.

An analysis that included 1503 patients from 34 trials for the second line of treatment for pancreatic cancer showed a median overall survival of 6 months among treated patients and 2.8 months for patients that underwent best supportive care but no chemotherapy ($p = 0.013$). Patients treated with either gemcitabine or platinum-based chemotherapy showed better outcomes when compared with other regimens, reported progression free survival was 4 months versus 1.6 months (p 0.059) and reported median overall survival was 6 months versus 5.3 months ($p = 0.1$), respectively [49].

Immunotherapy may represent an option in a very selected group of patients. A phase II trial showed promising activity of pembrolizumab, a PD-1 blocking antibody, in gastrointestinal cancers with deficiency of mismatch repair (dMMR) or high microsatellite instability (MSI-H) [50]. These finding lead to the site agnostic FDA approval for checkpoint inhibitors for dMMR/MSI-H tumors. ASCO 2018 guidelines for metastatic pancreatic cancer recommends dMMR/MSI-H testing to all patients with metastatic PC seeking for second line therapy, although this has modest real impact in PC, given that those abnormalities are present in only percent less than one percent of the patients [7].

Multiple gene testing with next generation sequencing test can lead to the identification of potentially target therapy that can be helpful for patients with metastatic PC, but there is no trial showing clear benefit of using this strategy. There are ongoing randomize trials exploring these options, making it a better option when available.

Stromal-depleting agents such as PEGPH20 have shown promising results in a phase 2 trial in untreated patients when combining with gemcitabine-Nab-paclitaxel in high hyaluronic acid population. These results have not been reproduced when PEGPH20 has been combined with FOLFIRINOX [51].

6. Conclusions

Pancreatic cancer is one of the most lethal malignancies among solid tumors and unfortunately most of the times it is diagnosed as a metastatic or unresectable disease with null chances of cure.

First systemic treatments for advanced pancreatic carcinoma were controversial in results and poor outcomes were historically reported.

In the 90's decade gemcitabine became the standard of care for advanced disease, with a mild improve in survival and in response rates. Looking to improve survival, response rate and quality of life several gemcitabine-based chemotherapy combinations were assessed in clinical trials but most of them failed in their primary end points. Despite, gemcitabine- erlotinib combination resulted in a positive trial in statistical terms when compared with gemcitabine alone, allowing to get FDA approval, the clinical significance was poor and currently it is not a recommended treatment as a first option.

No relevant advances were reported until 2011 when a phase 3 French clinical trial in advanced PC showed that FOLFIRINOX when compared with gemcitabine improved OS and response rate in advanced PC but with higher toxicity. 2 years later, in 2013, the publication of another phase clinical trial showed that gemcitabine plus nab-paclitaxel combination was superior than gemcitabine in terms of survival and responses, including patients older than 75 years and with worse performance status (0–2) than the French trial (0–1). Nevertheless, no phase 3 clinical trials have been conducted in order to answer which treatment is better than the other. Meta-analysis that have included both treatments show that apparently both regimens are similar in efficacy.

A recent publication showed that among BRCA-mutated advanced-PC adding olaparib as a maintenance treatment, in patients without disease progression after FOLFIRINOX, improves progression free survival but until now no benefit in overall survival has been reported.

Second-line therapy will depend on previous therapy and current performance status. Options for patients treated with gemcitabine-based regimens are 5-fluorouracil plus leucovorin plus either nanoliposomal irinotecan, irinotecan or oxaliplatin. Patients that were treated with first line FOLFIRINOX may benefit from a gemcitabine-based chemotherapy, but evidence from randomized trials is lacking. Other options like immunotherapy and targeted therapies yield benefit only in very selected cases, and it is still an area of research.

Conflict of interest

None of the authors received payments or any benefit for participating in this publication. This chapter has not been sponsored neither influenced for any pharmaceutical company, organization, or institution. Authors freely declare any personal potential conflict of interest that could be related or not with this manuscript.

Dr. Christian Caglevic: Honoraria: Andes Biotechnologies. Speaker: MSD, BMS, Lilly. Principal Investigator: MSD, GSK, Bayer, Boehringer Ingelheim, Astellas, Roche, Astra Zeneca, BMS, Novartis. Advisory and Consulting: MSD, BMS, Roche, Boehringer Ingelheim. Sponsored Educational Program (including travel, accommodations, and expenses): BMS, MSD, Roche.

Dr. Mauricio Mahave: no conflicts of interest.

Dr. Cristobal Sanhueza: Expert testimony: Tecnofarma. Travel-accommodations and expenses: Roche, Tecnofarma.

Dr. Luis Ubillos: Advisory and Consulting: Tecnofarma.

Author details

Christian Caglevic[1*], Mauricio Mahave[2], Cristobal Sanhueza[3] and Luis Ubillos[4]

1 Clinical Trials Unit, Cancer Research Department, Instituto Oncologico Fundacion Arturo Lopez Perez, Santiago, Chile

2 Medical Oncology Service, Instituto Oncologico Fundacion Arturo Lopez Perez, Santiago, Chile

3 Oncology Department, Facultad de Medicina, Clinica Alemana Santiago, Universidad del Desarrollo, Santiago, Chile

4 Medical Oncology, Hospital Britanico and Hospital de Clinicas UDELAR, Montevideo, Uruguay

*Address all correspondence to: christian.caglevic@falp.org

References

[1] Howlader N, Noone A, Krapcho M, et al. SEER Cancer Statistics Review, 1975-2016. Bethesda, MD: National Cancer Institute. 2019. Available from: https://seer.cancer.gov/csr/1975_2016/, based on November 2018 SEER data submission, posted to the SEER web site April 2019

[2] Paniccia A, Hosokawa P, Henderson W, et al. Characteristics of 10-year survivors of pancreatic ductal adenocarcinoma. JAMA Surgery. 2015;**150**(8):701-710. DOI: 10.1001/jamasurg.2015.0668

[3] Liu Q, Liao Q, Zhao Y. Chemotherapy and tumor microenvironment of pancreatic cancer. Cancer Cell International. 2017;**17**:68. DOI: 10.1186/s12935-017-0437-3. eCollection 2017

[4] Casper ES, Green MR, Kelsen DP, et al. Phase II trial of gemcitabine (2,2′-difluorodeoxycytidine) in patients with adenocarcinoma of the pancreas. Investigational New Drugs. 1994;**12**(1):29-34. DOI: 10.1007/BF00873232

[5] Moore MJ, Goldstein D, Hamm J, et al. Erlotinib plus gemcitabine compared with gemcitabine alone in patients with advanced pancreatic cancer: A phase III trial of the National Cancer Institute of Canada clinical trials group. Journal of Clinical Oncology. 2007;**25**(15):1960-1966. DOI: 10.1200/JCO.2006.07.9525

[6] Golan T, Sella T, O'Reilly EM, et al. Overall survival and clinical characteristics of BRCA mutation carriers with stage I/II pancreatic cancer. British Journal of Cancer. 2017;**116**(6):697-702. DOI: 10.1038/bjc.2017.19

[7] Macherla S, Laks S, Naqash A, et al. Emerging role of immune checkpoint blockade in pancreatic cancer. International Journal of Molecular Sciences. 2018;**19**(11):3505. DOI: 10.3390/ijms19113505

[8] Smith FP, Hoth DF, Levin B, et al. 5-fluorouracil, Adriamycin, and mitomycin-C (FAM) chemotherapy for advanced adenocarcinoma of the pancreas. Cancer. 1980;**46**(9): 2014-2018. DOI: 10.1002/1097-0142(19801101)46:9<2014::aid-cncr2820460920>3.0.co;2-d

[9] Cullinan SA, Moertel CG, Fleming TR. PhD; et al. a comparison of three chemotherapeutic regimens in the treatment of advanced pancreatic and gastric carcinoma. JAMA. 1985;**253**(14):2061. DOI: 10.1001/jama.1985.03350380077025

[10] Burris HA, Moore MJ, Andersen J, et al. Improvements in survival and clinical benefit with gemcitabine as first-line therapy for patients with advanced pancreas cancer: A randomized trial. Journal of Clinical Oncology. 1997;**15**(6):2403-2413. DOI: 10.1200/JCO.1997.15.6.2403

[11] Hu J, Zhao G, Wang H-X, et al. A meta-analysis of gemcitabine containing chemotherapy for locally advanced and metastatic pancreatic adenocarcinoma. Journal of Hematology & Oncology. 2011;**4**:11. Published online 2011 Mar 26. DOI: 10.1186/1756-8722-4-11

[12] Goncalves A, Gilabert M, Francois E, et al. BAYPAN study: A double-blind phase III randomized trial comparing gemcitabine plus sorafenib and gemcitabine plus placebo in patients with advanced pancreatic cancer. Annals of Oncology. 2012;**23**(11):2799-2805. DOI: 10.1093/annonc/mds135. Epub: 05 July 2012

[13] Ciliberto D, Botta C, Correale P, et al. Role of gemcitabine-based combination therapy in the management of advanced pancreatic cancer: A meta-analysis of randomised trials. European Journal of Cancer;**49**(3):593-603.

DOI: 10.1016/j.ejca.2012.08.019. Epub: 16 September 2012

[14] Ueno H, Ioka T, Ikeda M, et al. Randomized phase III study of gemcitabine plus S-1, S-1 alone, or gemcitabine alone in patients with locally advanced and metastatic pancreatic cancer in Japan and Taiwan: GEST study. Journal of Clinical Oncology. 2013;**31**(13):1640-1648. DOI: 10.1200/JCO.2012.43.3680. Epub: 01 April 2013

[15] Fjällskog M-LH, Lejonklou MH, Öberg KE, et al. Expression of molecular targets for tyrosine kinase receptor antagonists in malignant endocrine pancreatic tumors. Clinical Cancer Research. 2003;**9**(4):1469-1473

[16] Miyabayashi K, Ijichi H, Mohri D, et al. Erlotinib prolongs survival in pancreatic cancer by blocking gemcitabine-induced MAPK signals. Cancer Research. 2013;**73**(7):2221-2234. DOI: 10.1158/0008-5472.CAN-12-1453

[17] Boeck S, Vehling-Kaiser U, Waldschmidt D, et al. Erlotinib 150 mg daily plus chemotherapy in advanced pancreatic cancer: An interim safety analysis of a multicenter, randomized, cross-over phase III trial of the 'Arbeitsgemeinschaft Internistische Onkologie'. Anti-Cancer Drugs. 2010;**21**(1):94-100. DOI: 10.1097/CAD.0b013e32833123ed

[18] Caglevic C, Gallardo J, de la Torre M, et al. Recommendations for the management of pancreatic cancer type adenocarcinoma: A consensus statement reached during the 2015 Latin American Symposium on Gastroenterological Oncology. Revista Médica de Chile. 2016;**144**(10):1305-1318. DOI: 10.4067/s0034-98872016001000010

[19] Miksad RA, Schnipper L, Goldstein M. Does a statistically significant survival benefit of Erlotinib plus gemcitabine for advanced pancreatic cancer translate into clinical significance and value? Journal of Clinical Oncology;**25**(28):4506-4507. DOI: 10.1200/JCO.2007.13.0401

[20] Ychou M, Conroy T, Seitz JF, et al. An open label phase I study assessing the feasibility of the triple combination: Oxaliplatin plus irinotecan plus leucovorin/5-fluorouracil every 2 weeks in patients with advanced solid tumors. Annals of Oncology. 2003;**14**:481-489. DOI: 10.1093/annonc/mdg119

[21] Conroy T, Paillot B, Francois E, et al. Irinotecan plus oxaliplatin and leucovorin-modulated fluorouracil in advanced pancreatic cancer -- a Groupe Tumeurs digestives of the Fédération Nationale des Centres de Lutte Contre le cancer study. Journal of Clinical Oncology. 2005;**23**:1228-1236. DOI: 10.1200/JCO.2005.06.050

[22] Conroy T, Desseigne F, Ychou M, et al. FOLFIRINOX versus gemcitabine for metastatic pancreatic cancer. The New England Journal of Medicine. 2011;**364**(19):1817-1825. DOI: 10.1056/NEJMoa1011923

[23] Gourgou-Bourgade S, Bascoul-Mollevi C, Desseigne F, et al. Impact of FOLFIRINOX compared with gemcitabine on quality of life in patients with metastatic pancreatic cancer: Results from the PRODIGE 4/ACCORD 11 randomized trial. Journal of Clinical Oncology. 2013;**31**(1):23-29. DOI: 10.1200/JCO.2012.44.4869. Epub: 03 December 2012

[24] Tong H, Fan Z, Liu B, et al. The benefits of modified FOLFIRINOX for advanced pancreatic cancer and its induced adverse events: A systematic review and meta-analysis. Scientific Reports. 2018;**8**:8666. DOI: 10.1038/s41598-018-26811-9

[25] Mahaseth H, Brutcher E, Kauh J, et al. Modified FOLFIRINOX regimen with improved safety and maintained

efficacy in pancreatic adenocarcinoma. Pancreas. 2013;**42**(8):1311-1315. DOI: 10.1097/MPA.0b013e31829e2006

[26] Kundranda MN, Niu J. Albumin-bound paclitaxel in solid tumors: clinical development and future directions. Drug Design, Development and Therapy. 2015;**9**:3767-3777. Published 2015 Jul 24. DOI: 10.2147/DDDT.S88023

[27] Murakawa M, Aoyama T, Miyagi Y, et al. The impact of SPARC expression on the survival of pancreatic ductal adenocarcinoma patients after curative resection. Journal of Cancer. 2019;**10**(3):627-633. DOI: 10.7150/jca.28660

[28] Vaz J, Ansari D, Sasor A, Andersson R. SPARC: A potential prognostic and therapeutic target in pancreatic cancer. Pancreas. 2015;**44**(7):1024-1035. DOI: 10.1097/MPA.0000000000000409

[29] Frese KK, Neesse A, Cook N, et al. Nab-paclitaxel potentiates gemcitabine activity by reducing cytidine deaminase levels in a mouse model of pancreatic cancer. Cancer Discovery. 2012;**2**(3):260-269. DOI: 10.1158/2159-8290.CD-11-0242

[30] Von Hoff DD, Ramanathan RK, Borad MJ, et al. Gemcitabine plus nab-paclitaxel is an active regimen in patients with advanced pancreatic cancer: A phase I/II trial. Journal of Clinical Oncology. 2011;**29**(34):4548-4554. DOI: 10.1200/JCO.2011.36.5742

[31] Von Hoff DD, Ervin T, Arena FP, et al. Increased survival in pancreatic cancer with nab-paclitaxel plus gemcitabine. The New England Journal of Medicine. 2013;**369**(18):1691-1703. DOI: 10.1056/NEJMoa1304369

[32] Goldstein D, El-Maraghi RH, Hammel P, et al. nab-Paclitaxel plus gemcitabine for metastatic pancreatic cancer: Long-term survival from a phase III trial. Journal of the National Cancer Institute. 2015;**107**(2):pii: dju413. DOI: 10.1093/jnci/dju413. Print 2015 Feb

[33] Hammel P, Lacy J, Portales F, et al. Phase II LAPACT trial of nab-paclitaxel (nab-P) plus gemcitabine (G) for patients with locally advanced pancreatic cancer (LAPC). Journal of Clinical Oncology. 2018;**36** (4_suppl):204-204. DOI: 10.1200/JCO.2018.36.4_suppl.204

[34] Caglevic C, Panay S, Gallardo C, et al. Neoadjuvant treatment for nonmetastatic pancreatic cancer. In: Rodrigo L, editor. Advances in Pancreatic Cancer. Chapter 9. 2018. pp. 179-194. DOI: 10.5772/intechopen.75739

[35] Caglevic C, Panay S, Reyes FC, et al. Is neoadjuvant an option for the treatment of non-metastatic pancreatic cancer patients? Gastroenterol Hepatol Open Access. 2018;**9**(5):177-179. DOI: 10.15406/ghoa.2018.09.00321

[36] Pusceddu S, Ghidini M, Torchio M, et al. Comparative effectiveness of gemcitabine plus nab-paclitaxel and FOLFIRINOX in the first-line setting of metastatic pancreatic cancer: A systematic review and meta-analysis. Cancers (Basel). 2019;**11**(4):484. Published 2019 Apr 5. DOI: 10.3390/cancers11040484

[37] Golan T, Kanji Z, Epelbaum R, et al. Overall survival and clinical characteristics of pancreatic cancer in BRCA mutation carriers. British Journal of Cancer. 2014;**111**:1132-1138. DOI: 10.1038/bjc.2014.418

[38] Golan T, Hammel P, Reni M, et al. Maintenance Olaparib for Germline BRCA-mutated metastatic pancreatic cancer. The New England Journal of Medicine. 2019;**381**(4):317-327. DOI: 10.1056/NEJMoa1903387. Epub: 02 June 2019

[39] Wang-Gillam A, Li CP, Bodoky G, et al. Nanoliposomal irinotecan with fluorouracil and folinic acid in metastatic pancreatic cancer after previous gemcitabine-based therapy (NAPOLI-1): A global, randomised, open-label, phase 3 trial. Lancet. 2016;**387**(10018):545-557. DOI: 10.1016/S0140-6736(15)00986-1. Epub: 29 November 2015

[40] Wang-Gillam A, Hubnerb RA, Siveke JT, et al. NAPOLI-1 phase 3 study of liposomal irinotecan in metastatic pancreatic cancer: Final overall survival analysis and characteristics of long-term survivors. European Journal of Cancer. 2019;**108**:78-87. DOI: 10.1016/j.ejca.2018.12.007. Epub: 14 January 2019

[41] Zaniboni A, Aitini E, Barni S, et al. FOLFIRI as second-line chemotherapy for advanced pancreatic cancer: A GISCAD multicenter phase II study. Cancer Chemotherapy and Pharmacology. 2012;**69**(6):1641-1645. DOI: 10.1007/s00280-012-1875-1. Epub: 11 May 2012

[42] Gebbia V, Maiello E, Giuliani F, et al. Irinotecan plus bolus/infusional 5-fluorouracil and leucovorin in patients with pretreated advanced pancreatic carcinoma: A multicenter experience of the Gruppo Oncologico Italia Meridionale. American Journal of Clinical Oncology. 2010;**33**(5):461-464. DOI: 10.1097/COC.0b013e3181b4e3b0

[43] Sohal DPS, Kennedy EB, Khorana A, et al. Metastatic pancreatic cancer: ASCO clinical practice guideline update. Journal of Clinical Oncology. 2018;**36**(24):2545-2556. DOI: 10.1200/JCO.2018.78.9636. Epub: 23 May 2018

[44] Oettle H, Riess H, Stieler JM, et al. Second-line oxaliplatin, folinic acid, and fluorouracil versus folinic acid and fluorouracil alone for gemcitabine-refractory pancreatic cancer: Outcomes from the CONKO-003 trial. Journal of Clinical Oncology. 2014;**32**(23):2423-2429. DOI: 10.1200/JCO.2013.53.6995. Epub: 30 June 2014

[45] Gill S, Ko Y-J, Cripps C, et al. PANCREOX: A randomized phase III study of fluorouracil/leucovorin with or without oxaliplatin for second-line advanced pancreatic cancer in patients who have received gemcitabine-based chemotherapy. Journal of Clinical Oncology. 2016;**34**(32):3914-3920. DOI: 10.1200/JCO.2016.68.5776. Epub: 30 September 2016

[46] Nguyen KT, Kalyan A, Beasley HS, et al. Gemcitabine/nab-paclitaxel as second-line therapy following FOLFIRINOX in metastatic/advanced pancreatic cancer—Retrospective analysis of response. Journal of Gastrointestinal Oncology. 2017;**8**(3):556-565. DOI: 10.21037/jgo.2017.01.23

[47] Zhang H, Kellett C, Lambert P, Kim CA. Efficacy and tolerability of second-line nab-paclitaxel and gemcitabine after failure of first-line FOLFIRINOX for advanced pancreas cancer: A single-institution experience. Clinical Colorectal Cancer. 2018;**17**(3):e451-e456. DOI: 10.1016/j.clcc.2018.03.003. Epub: 08 March 2018

[48] Ahn DH, Krishna K, Blazer M, et al. A modified regimen of biweekly gemcitabine and nab-paclitaxel in patients with metastatic pancreatic cancer is both tolerable and effective: A retrospective analysis. Therapeutic Advances in Medical Oncology. 2017;**9**(2):75-82. DOI: 10.1177/1758834016676011. Epub: 02 November 2016

[49] Rahma OE, Duffy A, Liewehr DJ, et al. Second-line treatment in advanced pancreatic cancer: A comprehensive analysis of published clinical trials. Annals of Oncology.

2013;**24**(8):1972-1979. DOI: 10.1093/annonc/mdt166. Epub: 12 May 2013

[50] Le DT, Uram JN, Wang H, et al. PD-1 blockade in tumors with mismatch-repair deficiency. The New England Journal of Medicine. 2015;**372**(26):2509-2520. DOI: 10.1056/NEJMoa1500596

[51] Mohammad A. Advanced pancreatic cancer: The standard of care and new opportunities. Oncology Reviews. 2018;**12**:370. DOI: 10.4081/oncol.2018.370

Chapter 6

An Overview of Pancreatic Neuroendocrine Tumors

Neha Sharma and Deepti Sharma

Abstract

Pancreatic neuroendocrine tumors are a group of endocrine tumors that constitute 7% of all pancreatic neoplasms. They can be benign or malignant. Their presentation can vary from slow growing, non infiltrative, indolent masses to rapidly progressing, highly aggressive, metastasizing tumors. In the past, there was paucity of scientific data available about the diagnosis and treatment strategy of these neoplasms but in recent years, ongoing research has inferred much data regarding classification, prognostic stratification and therapy of pancreatic neuroendocrine tumors. In this chapter we will discuss epidemiology, clinical presentation and classification, diagnosis and management of these tumors. We will also deliberate about the latest developments in treatment of pancreatic neuroendocrine tumors with focus on recent studies done on this topic.

Keywords: pancreatic neuroendocrine tumors, pancreatic NET, GEP-NET, Gastroenteropancreatic tumor

1. Introduction

Neuro-endocrine tumors constitute 0.5% of all malignancies [1]. Gastro-entero-pancreatic neuro-endocrine tumors (GEP-NET) originate from neuro-endocrine cells of the embryological gut and they constitute a group of heterogeneous tumors that demonstrate divergent tumor biology, different diagnostic behavior, management principles and tumor-patient outcomes [2].

2. Incidence and epidemiology

GEP-NET comprises 2% of all gastrointestinal tumors [3]. Pancreatic neuroendocrine tumors (PNETs) are one of the most common neuroendocrine tumors [4]. But they are relatively rare tumors and comprise about 7% of all cancers that occur in the pancreas [5]. According to The American Cancer Society's estimates for 2020, about 4,032 people in the United States will be diagnosed with pancreatic NET.[8]

With better imaging modalities coming into play, the incidence of pancreatic NETs is increasing over the years as they are often found incidentally when radiological tests such as CT or MRI scans are done for other diseases. There has also been increased sensitivity of lab tests that have escalated the ability to distinguish these tumors from other malignancies. The increased prevalence over the past few decades, is attributed to multifactorial causes mainly as a consequence of increased awareness and improved diagnostic technique [6]. It is estimated that nowadays almost 50% of PNET diagnoses are incidentalomas [7]. An aging population and heightened awareness of the disease have also contributed to an increase in the detection of incidentalomas [8].

Majority of pNET are sporadic, i.e. non inherited while 10–30% pNET are associated with a genetic syndrome like multiple endocrine neoplasia (MEN) type 1, which is most commonly associated with it [9]. Other rare genetic conditions include MEN4, Von Hippel–Lindau disease, neurofibromatosis 1 (von Recklinghausen's syndrome), and tuberous sclerosis, which are linked to genetic type pNET [10].

There is no gender predilection for pNET although some studies have suggested a slight preponderance for men. These tumors can present at any age but the incidence of sporadic tumors rises from fifth decade and peaks around 80s [11].

3. Classification and staging

In the past NETs were classified based upon the site of origin in embryological gut as foregut, midgut and hindgut tumors. It has been rather challenging to classify these tumors due to their heterogeneity, difference in their morphology, clinical presentation, molecular biology, hormone profile and treatment response.

Clinically these tumors have been classified as functioning and non functioning tumors. In 2007 WHO introduced a new classification system for neuroendocrine tumors which categorized them according to tumor's proliferation indices like mitotic index or Ki67 score as well differentiated tumors and poorly differentiated carcinomas [12]. In 2010 it also included histopathological features as a criteria for classification apart from proliferation indices, which lead to revision of the existing guidelines and NETs were further divided into three grades based upon ENETS classification (**Table 1**) [14]. Well differentiated tumors comprised of grade 1 and grade 2 NET, while poorly differentiated tumors were grade 3 NET also described as neuroendocrine carcinoma (NEC). The difference between the two has been illustrated in **Table 2** [14].

In 2017, the classification was re-revised to include NET grade1, 2 and 3 in the well differentiated category and the poorly differentiated category was NEC grade 3. See **Table 3** [15].

European neuroendocrine society has also devised a staging for GEP-NET. American cancer society has included tumor resectability as classification criteria (**Figure 1**) [17].

Mixed adenoneuroendocrine carcinoma (MANEC) of pancreas are a group of extremely rare tumors, with incidence approximately 0.2% and only a few cases are reported in literature [18]. They have both adenocarcinoma and neuroendocrine components with each component accounting for more than 30% of the tumor [19]. Due to rarity of this, tumor the clinical behavior is not studied much. It has been proposed that the treatment should depend on the aggressiveness of the cell type of the tumor [20]. In various cases studied, surgery has been considered as the first line of treatment for resectable tumors. Post operative treatment includes adjuvant chemotherapy and/or radiotherapy [21].

Well differentiated net	Ki67 index	Mitotic index
NET G1	<=2%	<2/hpf
NET G2	3–20%	2–20/hpf
Poorly differentiated net		
NEC	>20%	>20/hpf

Table 1.
Who classification 2010 [13].

Characteristics	NET G3	NEC
Pathological differentiation	Well differentiated	Poorly differentiated
Ki 67 index	>20% (usually 30–55%)	>20%(usually 50%)
Mitotic index	>20/hpf	>20/hpf
necrosis	Rare	present
Genetic syndrome MEN1, VHL	occasionally	rare
Functionality	occasionally	rare
Neuroendocrine marker expression	positive	weak
Somatostatin receptor scintigraphy uptake	strong	weak
Loss of ATR x and DAXX protein expression	present	rare
Abnormal p53, SMAD4 and Rb expression	rare	present
Response to platinum agents	worse	better
Prognosis	Relatively good	poor

Table 2.
The difference between NET Grade3 and NEC grade3 [15].

Well differentiated net	Ki67 index	Mitotic index
NET G1	<3%	<2/hpf
NET G2	3–20%	2–20/hpf
NET G3	>20%	>20/hpf
Poorly differentiated net		
NEC	>20%	>20/hpf

Table 3.
Who classification 2017 [13].

AJCC Staging Classification		ENETS Staging Classification	
T1	Tumor limited to the pancreas, <2 cm	T1	Tumor limited to the pancreas, <2 cm
T2	Tumor limited to the pancreas, >2 cm	T2	Tumor limited to the pancreas, 2-4 cm
T3	Tumor extends beyond the pancreas, but not involving the celiac axis or SMA	T3	Tumor limited to the pancreas, >4 cm, or invading duodenum or CBD
T4	Tumor involves the celiac axis or SMA	T4	Tumor invades adjacent structures
N0	No regional LN metastasis	N0	No regional LN metastasis
N1	Regional LN metastasis	N1	Regional LN metastasis
M0	No distant metastasis	M0	No distant metastasis
M1	Distant metastasis	M1	Distant metastasis

Stage	T	N	M	Stage	T	N	M
IA	T1	N0	M0	I	T1	N0	M0
IB	T2	N0	M0	IIA	T2	N0	M0
IIA	T3	N0	M0	IIB	T3	N0	M0
IIB	T1-3	N1	M0	IIIA	T4	N0	M0
III	T4	N0-1	M0	IIIB	Any T	N1	M0
IV	Any T	Any N	M1	IV	Any T	Any N	M1

	ENETS I	ENETS II	ENETS III	ENETS IV
AJCC I	25	59	0	0
AJCC II	0	4	37	0
AJCC III	0	0	18	0
AJCC IV	0	0	0	282

CBD = common bile duct; LN = lymph node; SMA = superior mesenteric artery.

Figure 1.
Comparison of TNM classification of pancreatic NENs according to ENETS versus UICC/AJCC (TNM classification) [16].

4. Etiopathogenesis

4.1 Cellular biology of net

As such pNETs were classically thought to arise from pancreatic islet cells or the islets of Langerhans, hence the term islet cell tumors was coined [22]. Islet cells are the endocrine cells of the pancreas and they constitute 1–2% of total pancreatic mass. They are therefore distinct from the exocrine cells, from which pancreatic ductal adenocarcinomas arise. They are composed of various cell types and responsible for secretion of hormones like beta cells (insulin), alpha cells (glucagon), delta cells (somatostatin), and PP cells (pancreatic polypeptide) [23]. However, current theory says that pNETs in fact arise from the APUD (amine precursor uptake and decarboxylation) cells [24]. The presence of neurosecretory granules is the characteristic feature of APUD cells and these neurosecretory granules have autocrine, paracrine and neuromodulatory functions, in addition to the endocrine property. These cells are thought to originate in the embryologic neural crest, but more recent research suggests that they originate in the embryologic endoderm [25].

The most common genes involved in pancreatic neuroendocrine tumors are mentioned in **Table 4**.

Other specific genes suggested to be implicated in the etiopathogenesis of NETs include BIN1, Serpine 10, BST2, IGFBP3, LCK, MET, fibronectin, PDGF, IGF- 1, fibroblast growth factor, TGF-alpha and–beta, EGFR, and stem cell factor receptor [27].

Multiple studies have elucidated the underlying genetic mechanism regarding molecular development and progression of these tumors but still much remains unexplored in this area. Loss of chromosomes 3q, 6pq, and 10 pq, and gains of 5q, 12a, 18q, and 20q is associated with malignant behavior in these tumors [28]. In tumors less than 2 cm in size, it has been observed that Chromosome 1 and 11q loss with gain of 9q is associated with genetic instability [29].

4.2 Olecular pathology of PNET and its role in prognosis

Most recent advancements in assessment of pancreatic NET is the development of microRNA profiling which corresponds to various proliferation indices and also propensity of tumor to cause local spread and distant metastasis [30]. MicroRNA are non-coding RNA sequences having length of 21–25 nucleotides. They regulate genes at post translational level [31]. They can act as oncogenes or tumor suppressor genes and play a significant role in proliferation of tumors or their dissemination [32]. They can act as diagnostic as well as a prognostic marker.

There is very limited data available regarding microRNA profiling of pNET. In one large study done on pancreatic NET, 28 different miRs have been shown to

Gene	Prevalence in PNET	Prevalence in PDAC
MEN1	44%	0%
ATRX/DAXX	43%	0%
mTOR	15%	0.8%
TP53	3%	85%
KRAS	0%	100%
CDKN2A	0%	25%
TGFBR1/SMAD3/SMAD4	0%	38%

Table 4.
Common genes in pancreatic neuroendocrine tumors vs. pancreatic adenocarcinoma [26, 27].

be differentially expressed with 18 of them being higher expressed and 10 lower expressed as compared to healthy pancreatic tissue [33]. There is a higher expression of miR-103, miR-107 and miR-193b and lower expression of let-7 miR and miR-155 in pancreatic neuroendocrine neoplasias [34]. Tumor proliferation is denoted by expression levels of miR-196a, miR-21 and miR-642 while miR-210 and miR-21 seem to correlate with metastatic disease and tumor recurrence is predicted by expression of both miR-196a and miR-27b [35, 36].

Circulating tumor cell count also plays an important role in delineating the prognostic value of pNETs, especially before and during the treatment. Liquid biopsy is emerging as a newer and more profound biomarker test which provides valid cytochemical, morphological, pathological and molecular information regarding response of anti tumor therapy for pNET [37]. Circulating tumor cells (CTC) are shed from the primary or metastatic component of the tumor and they are evaluated by liquid biopsy [38]. CTC are considered as prognosticators in many solid malignancies but their role in neuroendocrine tumors was highlighted first by Khan et al. in 2011 [39] patients with advanced NETs who were starting either systemic or local therapy were enrolled. It was found that patients with one or more circulating tumor cells (CTC) were more likely to have worse progression free and overall survival.

Further placental growth factor (PIGF) is also evaluated as a prospective biomarker in NET. pIGF is a derivative of VEGF, which shows increased expression in NETs. It was found that PlGF levels were elevated in pNET samples and serum as compared to control pancreatic tissue and control serum. It was concluded that elevated PIGF levels are seen in pNET and it has also been projected that increase PIGF levels correlate with shorter time to progression [40].

5. Clinical presentation

Since non functional pNET represent up to 90% of PanNETs, they present with high hormone levels without symptoms. However, upto 60% of these patients have a metastatic disease at diagnosis, while 21% present with a locally advanced disease [41].

Non specific symptoms of pNET include abdominal pain, weight loss, or mass effect related to the pancreatic tumor or to the distant spread. Less frequently it is associated with complaints of jaundice, hemorrhage from tumors, and a palpable mass. Symptoms often do not appear until metastases develop [42].

Usually endocrine tumors of the pancreas present with typical symptoms due to hormonal hypersecretion, such as insulinoma, gastrinoma, VIP-oma, glucagonoma and somatostatinoma. In upto 40%-50, cases may present as non-functioning tumors or secrete pancreatic polypeptide (PP) and neurotensin [43]. The various pancreatic NET subtypes with their incidence, clinical presentation and survival are mentioned below (**Table 5**).

6. Diagnosis

6.1 Biochemical

Chromogranin A is a secretory glycoprotein present in neurosecretory granules of pancreatic NET. Majority of pNET show elevated chromogranin A levels. The sensitivity depends upon the tumor burden and the levels of chromogranin A are directly correlated with the prognosis of the patient. In insulinomas elevated

Tumor/Syndrome	Incidence	Associated Symptoms	Malignancy	Associated peptide	Survival
Insulinoma [45]/ Hypoglycemia Syndrome	1–4 per million per year	Confusion, sweating, dizziness, weakness, relief with eating	10% patients develop metastasis	insulin	Complete resection leads to cure
Gastrinoma [46]/zollinger ellison syndrome	1–2 per million per year	Diarrhea with or without severe peptic ulcertion	60% patients develop metastasis, likelihood correlated with size of primary	gastrin	Complete resection leads to 10 year survival 90%
Glucagonoma [47]	0.1 per million per year	Weight loss, diabetes mellitus,necrolytic migratory erythema	60% patients develop metastasis	glucagon	Most favorable prognosis with complete resection, even in cases with liver metastasis
VIPoma [48]/ verner morrison syndrome	0.05% to 2.0%	Profuse watery diarrhea, hypokalemia, hypochlorhydria	70%patients develop metastasis Usually at diagnosis	Vasoactive intestinal polypeptide	Complete resection associated with 5 year survival 95%, With metastasis 60%
Somatostatinoma [49]	1 in 40 million	Cholelithiasis, weight loss, steatorrhea, diarrhea, diabetes mellitus, achlorhydria	50% patients develop metastasis	Somatostatin	Complete resection associated with 5 year survival 95%,, With metastasis 60%
ACTHoma [50]	<0.1	Cushing syndroma		ACTH	
PTHrPoma/ pNET causing hypercalcemia [32]	<0.1	Symptoms due to raised Ca levels		PTHrP	
GRFoma [32]	<0.1	acromegaly		GRF	
Non syndromic pancreatic neuroendocrine syndrome [32]		Symptoms due to pancreatic mass or liver metastasis	50% patients develop metastasis		Complete resection associated with 5 year survival 50%

Table 5.
Incidence, clinical presentation and survival of pancreatic NET subgroups [27–32, 44].

chromogranin A levels are rare. Other serologic markers include neuronal serum enolase, human chorionic gonadotropin, and pancreatic polypeptide, which are elevated in 20–40% of PNETs. (See **Table 6**) [52].

When any NET is suspected then fasting gut hormones such as chromogranin B, pancreatic polypeptide and urinary 5HIAA (a breakdown product of serotonin) are also useful baseline tests. False positive chromogranin A levels are caused due to treatment with a proton pump inhibitor, Parkinson's disease, hypertension, glucocorticoids, renal failure and atrophic gastritis, while various dietary factors and drugs can cause an elevated urinary 5HIAA [53].

Additional blood tests for secreted peptides can be useful if a clinical syndrome is suspected and calcium, prolactin and parathyroid hormones should be tested in possible MEN1 cases. For Nonfunctioning pNETs, pancreatic polypeptide is a useful test. For insulinomas the gold standard diagnostic tool is supervised fasting with serial blood glucose analysis. Diagnosis requires the fulfillment of Whipple's triad of hypoglycemia, symptoms and correction of symptoms with glucose, in the presence of non-suppressed insulin levels. Factitious hypoglycemia due to administration of insulin or sulfonylureas must be ruled out [54].

6.2 Radiological

Cross sectional imaging plays an important role in the workup of PNETs by characterizing the primary tumor and determining the extent of disease. Location of the tumor and its spread can be delineated by the use of multimodality imaging which includes computed tomography (CT), MRI and various nuclear medicine scans. Endoscopic ultrasound (EUS), digital subtraction angiography and venous sampling can also be used [55]. The sensitivity of CT and MRI is more than 80% for the detection of PNETs which is more sensitive than an octreotide-based scintigraphic scans [56].

EUS acts as an indispensable accompaniment to CT or MRI and has superior resolution. For tumors with size as small as 2 mm, EUS shows sensitivity of more than 90% and when combined with cross sectional imaging the sensitivity reaches upto 100%. Addition of EUS is recommended when cross-sectional imaging fails to define the pancreatic mass, when the location of primary cannot be delineated or biopsy is needed to confirm the diagnosis before commencing the treatment [57].

Syndrome	Test	Result
Gastrinoma	Fasting gastrin Gastrin secretion studies	Raised basal serum gastrin, High gastric acid secretion
Insulinoma	Fasting Insulin, Glucose, C peptide (sulfonyl urea screen negative)	Raised fasting insulin/glucose ratio, proinsulin or c peptide
Glucagonoma	Fasting gut hormones, ski biopsy	Raised serum pancreatic glucagons and enteroglucagon
VIPoma	Fasting gut hormone	Raised fasting VIP
Ppoma	Fasting gut hormone	Raised fasting pancreatic polypeptide
Somatostatinoma	Fasting gut hormone	Raised fasting somatostatin
All NET	Serum chromogranin	Raised chromogranin A
Ectopic hormones	GHRH, ACTH, HCG-alpha and beta	Raised but low incidence

Table 6.
Biochemical tests for pNET [33, 51].

Well Differentiated Net [63]	Poorly Differentiated Net [64]
• "organoid" arrangements of the tumor cells • solid, nested, trabecular, or ribbon-like/gyriform, tubulo-acinar/pseudoglandular and mixed pattern • Uniform cells with round to oval nuclei, coarsely granular, 'salt and pepper' chromatin • pale to moderately eosinophilic cytoplasm • Has neurosecretory granules • Necrosis absent	• Sheets or nests of atypical cells • pleomorphic, hyperchromatic nuclei and abundant mitotic figures • 'Salt and pepper' appearance of chromatin is absent • Necrosis often present • small cell (molding nuclei, scant cytoplasm) or large cell (abundant amphophilic cytoplasm

Table 7.
Histopathological features of well and poorly differentiated tumors.

Since NETs have high levels of somatostatin receptor 2 (SSTR2) expression, Functional imaging comes into play in these tumors. For tumors lacking SSTR2, like insulinomas and poorly differentiated tumors, it is less useful [58]. It is used to detect primary tumors or metastatic disease which is not readily seen on cross-sectional imaging. Also, the uptake can predict response to octreotide analogs [59].

Indium-111 (111In) pentetreotide scan (Octreoscan) is a readily available nuclear scan that is effective at identifying nonfunctional PNETs, glucagonomas, and gastrinomas [60]. Although High-resolution positron emission tomography (PET) in combination with CT is superior in detecting small tumors and identifying occult metastases as compared to 111In pentetreotide. For identifying well-differentiated NETs, Octreoscan appears more sensitive than (18) FDG-PET, whereas (18) FDG-PET demonstrates superior sensitivity for poorly-differentiated NETs [61].

Somatostatin receptors are overexpressed in a proportion of NETs and Somatostatin receptor scintigraphy (SSRS) is useful in detecting these tumors. There are five subtypes of SSTR and 80% of pNETs, excluding insulinomas, express SSTR-2. Less than half of insulinomas express SSRT-2, therefore Single-photon emission computed tomography (SPECT) has sensitivity of 50% when combined with SSRS. In gastrinomas, VIPomas, glucagonomas and nonfunctional tumors SSRS combined with SPECT has a diagnostic sensitivity of 75% [20].

Currently both 18F-FDG PET/CT and 68Gallium (Ga)-labeled somatostatin analog PET/CTs such as 68Ga-DOTATOC or 68Ga-DOTATATE PET/CTs are used. FDGPET use is limited to poorly differentiated NETs, as well differentiated NETs are not FDG avid. It may also be used to demonstrate aggressive behavior or heterogeneity between lesions in a single patient. 68Ga-labeled somatostatin analog PETs have been shown to be superior to CT or SSRS in sensitivity and specificity, for detecting an unknown primary, staging at diagnosis, and for follow-up [62].

6.3 Histopathology

They can be classified as well differentiated and poorly differentiated NET. the major differences are elaborated further (**Table 7**).

7. DIfferential diagnosis

- Acinar cell carcinoma: It can be differentiated from pNET as it has granular PAS positive cytoplasm, BCL10, trypsin, chymotrypsin positive, Synaptophysin and chromogranin positivity <25% while pNET is PAS negative,

BCL10, trypsin, chymotrypsin negative and Synaptophysin or chromogranin positivity over 25% [65].

- Solid-pseudopapillary neoplasm: It has pseudopapillary architecture, Chromogranin focal to negative, Galectin 3,Vimentin, CD10, Nuclear beta catenin positive while pNET has no pseudopapillary architecture, Chromogranin strongly positive, Galectin 3,Vimentin, CD10, Nuclear beta catenin negative [65].

- Pancreatoblastoma: It shows Trypsin, chymotrypsin positive, Chromogranin, synaptophysin scattered positive, Islet polypeptide markers negative or very focal while Trypsin, chymotrypsin negative, Chromogranin or synaptophysin widespread staining, Islet polypeptide markers frequently positive in pNET [65]

Insulinoma [27]: the differential diagnosis includes conditions with increased insulin levels in blood

- Persistent hyperinsulinemic hypoglycemia of infancy (PHHI)
- Sulfonylurea-induced hypoglycemia
- Insulin autoimmune hypoglycemia
- Post-gastric bypass hypoglycemia
- Noninsulinoma pancreatogenous hypoglycemia syndrome (NIPHS)
- Non-islet-cell tumors that secrete insulin-like growth factors (IGF)
- Factitious use of insulin

Glucagonoma [66].

- Acrodermatitis Enteropathica
- Bacteremia
- Cirrhosis
- Non functioning neuroendocrine tumor
- Paraneoplastic Syndromes
- Pediatric Pellagra
- Psoriasis
- Type 1 and 2 Diabetes Mellitus

8. Management

Multidisciplinary teams (MDTs) have an important role in deciding the treatment of these tumors as they are slightly rare.

Treatment options range from curative surgery to palliation with medical therapies including somatostatin analogs, chemotherapy and targeted treatments [67].

Conservative management is indicated for incidentalomas, i.e. the tumors which are small, non functional and asymptomatic [68]. Although it is a controversy whether small nonfunctional tumors of under 2 cm should be resected, when they are likely to have less metastatic potential, but a more aggressive surgical approach is recommended for tumors over 2 cm [69].

8.1 Surgery

Surgery is the only curative treatment option and should be considered in all patients with localized disease as it not only cures the mass related symptoms but also the hormone related effects. Such patients should have their surgery carried out at specialist hepatopancreatobiliary centers. Surgery can be done for curative treatment like radical excision or palliative treatment that aims for symptomatic relief. It can also be used for surgical treatment of complications. The 5-year overall survival rate of resected PNETs is significantly greater than unresected ones, ranging from 77% to 46% [70]. Unfortunately, pancreatic surgery shows significant mortality, ranging from 1% to 10% [71] and morbidity. The perioperative and long-term complications include diabetes, pancreatic exocrine impairment in up to 50–60% patients, even in high volume centers [72, 73].

Careful observation and wait and watch policy can be employed for small non functioning pNET which helps in not only avoiding the pancreatic surgery but also helps curb the operation related complications, as most of the small NF-PanNETs are indolent despite a chance of 10% of nodal involvement [74, 75].

According to the updated ENET guidelines patients having NF-PanNETs ≤2 cm can be safely managed conservatively.

Indications of non operative approach:

- the presence of G1-low G2 tumor
- Tumor localized to pancreatic head
- no signs of malignancy at imaging.

In patients with G2 NF-PanNETs greater than or equal to 2 cm, surgery should be recommended. Other factors to be taken into consideration include patient's age, comorbidities, surgical risk, the tumor site, and desire for surgical intervention.

In cases of surveillance, EUS and MRI should be mandatory and to be repeated every 6 months (12 months if no changes are discovered). If an increase of 0.5 cm (or more) in the size of the lesion is seen on the imaging then the patient should be reevaluated for surgery [9].

The studies comparing observation with surgery in pNET are as follows:(**Table 8**).

In contrast to the ENETS guidelines, the American National Comprehensive Cancer Network (NCCN) guidelines recommend surgery to be done in a pNET bigger than 1 cm. Observation is indicated incidentally discovered, low-grade NF-PanNETs smaller than 1 cm. Additional factors for conservative management include the surgical risk, the tumor site, and the patient comorbidities, especially when dealing with small asymptomatic tumor [80]. NCCN states that more aggressive approach (routine surgery) is recommended in tumors greater than 1 cm as some small (<2 cm) high-grade tumors demonstrate frankly malignant behavior (9% to 39%) [81].

Study	No. of patients	Protocol	Result
Sadot et al. [76]	Incidentally discovered, sporadic, small (<3 cm), stage I–II PanNET 464 patients	Observation 104 patients vs. surgery 77 patients	No diff in os in both groups
Rosenberg et al. [77]	Incidentally discovered non functional pNET	Observation 15 patients vs. surgery 20 patients	Incidentally discovered NF-PNETs <2 cm in size can be observed safely with serial imaging.
Regenet et al. [78]	80 patients Non functional pNET	Observation 66 patients vs. 10 surgery	Tumor size has great impact on malignancy. he cutoff of 2 cm of malignancy used for small NF-PNETs could be decreased to 1.7 cm to select patients more accurately.
Zhang et al. [79]	Small non functioning pNET 249 patients`	Observation 56 vs. surgery 193	Resection of nonfunctioning PNETs over 1.5 cm is independently and significantly associated with a longer survival

Table 8.
Studies comparing observation versus surgery in small pNET.

8.2 Systemic therapy

In patients with resectable PanNETs, surgery with curative intent (that is, R0 or margins that are microscopically free of tumor) remains the treatment of choice. Unfortunately, as the majority of patients with PanNETs either present with metastatic disease or have disease recurrence within 2 years of surgery, effective systemic therapies are also needed [82].

8.3 Somatostatin analogs

Somatostatin analogs remain the cornerstone in treatment of advanced neuroendocrine tumors.

Long acting octrotide, lanreotide which bind both SSTR2 and SSTR5 and pasireotide which binds to SSTR1, 3, and 5 are currently approved for clinical use [83].

Trials studying the role of somatostatin analogues (**Table 9**).

Study	No. of patients	Protocol	Result
PROMID TRIAL [84]	85 patients with well-differentiated NETs	long-acting octreotide (n = 42) vs. placebo (n = 43)	Octreotide LAR significantly lengthens time to tumor progression compared with placebo. Ttp octreotide 14.3 month vs. placebo 6 month
CLARINET TRIAL [85]	204 patients with advanced, G1/G2 differentiated, nonfunctioning, somatostatin receptor–positive NETs	Lanreotide(n = 101) vs. placebo(n = 103)	Better PFS with lanreotide Median PFS lanreotide(32.8 month) vs. placebo(18 month)

Table 9.
Studies showing role of somatostatin analogues in pNET.

The use of pasireotide, a somatostatin analog was evaluated in a phase III randomized trial targeting SSTR5, in octreotide-resistant patients. It demonstrated no difference in the response rate (RR) compared with long-acting octreotide. The trial was stopped prematurely [86].

Chan et al., studied 1022 patients in 18 trials using more than 30 mg octreotide or 120 mg lanreotide over 28 days in a meta-analysis in 2017 [87]. Pasireotide has shown a more potent antiproliferative effect as compared to octreotide in preclinical data from NCI-H727 cells and from pancreatic NET primary cell cultures [88].

A similar study conducted by Cives et al. recently showed that pasireotide LAR provides better tumor control efficacy (PFS 11 months), when used as first-line therapy in patients with advanced NET [89]. Further, in patients with functionally active advanced GEP-NETs, pasireotide provided an improved tumor control rate at 6 months compared to octreotide [50]. In 160 patients with progressive grade 1 through 2 pancreatic NETs, the COOPERATE-2 trial tested the combination of everolimus and pasireotide vs. everolimus. It was seen that both overall and progression-free survival were similar in both arms (16.8 months vs. 16.6 months), although response rates were higher in the experimental arm [90].

Study Design	No of patients	protocol	Result
Kulke et al. 2008 [91] Phase 2	Out of 109 patients, pancreatic endocrine tumor, n = 66	oral sunitinib	ORR) in pancreatic endocrine tumor patients was 16.7% SD68% MEDIAN PFS 81% (1-year survival)
Raymond et al. [92] Phase 3	171 patients	Placebo (n = 85) vs. sunitinib(n = 86)	Median PFS was 11.4 months in the sunitinib group as compared with 5.5 months in the placebo group. objective response rate was 9.3% in the sunitinib group versus 0% in the placebo group
Yao et al. [93] Phase 2	200 patients	Everolimus(n = 115) Everolimus + octreotide LAR(n = 85)	Median PFS 9.6 months Median PFS 16.7 mo.
Yao et al. [94] Phase 2	30 patients	Everolimus + octreotide LAR	Median PFS 12.5 mo.
Yao et al. [95] Phase 3	410 patients	Everolimus (n = 207) vs. placebo (n = 203)	Median PFS 11 mo vs. 4.6 mo.
Duran et al. [96] Phase 2	15 patients	temsirolimus	median TTP 6 months and 1-year OS rate 71.5%
Hobday et al. [97] Phase 2	43 patients	sorafenib	Median PFS 6 month
Phan et al. [98] Phase 2	29 patients	Pazopanib + octreotide LAR	Median PFS 11.7 months

Table 10.
Studies showing the role of targeted therapy in treatment of pNET.

Study Design	No of patients	protocol	Result
Broder et al. [63] Phase 2	52	streptozocin	A significant increase in 1-year survival rate and a doubling of median survival were shown for the responders as compared with the nonresponders
Moertel et al. [101] Phase 3	84	Streptozocin (n = 42) vs. streptozocin plus 5FU (n = 86)	Median OS was 26.5 months in the streptozocin plus 5FU group as compared with 16.5 months in the streptozocin group
Moertel et al. [102] Phase 3	105	Streptozocin/Doxo(n = 38) Streptozocin +5FU(n = 34) Chlorozotocin (n = 33)	Median OS 26.4 months Median OS 16.8 mo. Median OS 18 mo
Moertel et al. [103] Phase 2	14	Cisplatin + etoposide	
Turner et al. [104] Phase 2	47	Cisplatin/5-FU/ streptozocin	
Ramanathan et al. [105]	50	Dacarbazine	median OS 19.3 months
Bajetta et al. [106]	27	Capecitabine/oxaliplatin	
Kulke et al. [107] Phase 2	11	Temozolomide/thalidomide	Median OS 24 months
Chan et al. [108]	15	Bevacizumab Plus Temozolomide	median overall survival was 41.7 months for pancreatic NETs
Chan et al. [109]	43	Temozolamide and everolimus	the median progression-free survival duration was 15.4 months. Median overall survival was not reached
BETTER trial [110]	34	Bevacizumab with 5-FU/ streptozocin	Median PFS 23.7 months OS rate at 24 months was 88%.

Table 11.
Studies showing role of cytotoxic chemotherapy in pNET.

8.4 Targeted therapy

Molecular targeted therapies have emerged as a promising treatment modality for patients with well-differentiated PNETs in which disease progression is seen on a somatostatin analog or who are on best supportive care. Randomized studies have shown an improvement in PFS but not OS. Currently, sunitinib and everolimus are approved for use in PNETs (**Table 10**).

8.5 Cytotoxic chemotherapies

Much of the focus on treatment over the past half century has been on the use of conventional cytotoxic agents such as streptozocin [99] and temozolomide [100]. Sunitinib and everolimus are approved for use in PNETs (**Table 11**).

8.6 Peptide receptor radionuclide therapy (PRRT)

Majority of neuroendocrine tumors show increased level expression of somatostatin receptors (SSRs) 2 and 5 on the tumor cell surface and it forms the basis

Study	No. of Patients	Radioligand	Result
Valkema et al. [114]	58	90Y-DOTATOC	PFS 29 months OS 17 months
Kwekkeboom et al. [115]	310	177Lu-DOTATATE	PFS 33 months OS 46 months
Bushnell et al. [116]	90	90Y-DOTATOC	PFS 16 months OS 27 months
Cwikla et al. [117]	58	90Y-DOTATATE	PFS 17 months OS 22 months
Pfeifer et al. [118]	53	90Y-DOTATOC	PFS 29 months OS - months
Bodei et al. [119]	39	177Lu-DOTATATE	PFS 36 months OS - months
Ezziddin et al. [120]	74	177Lu-DOTATATE	PFS 26 months OS 55 months

Table 12.
Various retrospective studies have been conducted on PRRT.

of not only functional imaging but also tumor directed therapies like somatostatin analogues [111]. Beyond somatostatin analogues, PRRT, which is described as peptide receptor radioligand therapy or targeted radiotherapy using radiolabeled somatostatin analogs is emerging as an effective treatment modality in metastatic, well-differentiated, grade 1 and 2 GEP-NET [112]. Yttrium, a high-energy β particle emitter and Lutetium, a β and γ particle emitter with lower tissue penetration are most commonly studied radioligands [113] (**Table 12**).

131I-metaiodobenzylguanidine (131I-MIBG) therapy has shown promise in in MIBG positive metastatic neuroendocrine tumors, in addition to radiolabeled somatostatin analogs [121].

The toxicities associated with PRRT include myelosuppression and nephrotoxicity, both of which are reversible, acute pain due to radiation edema and nausea and vomiting, associated with the use of amino acids to reduce the risk of nephrotoxicity and very rarely myelodysplastic syndrome.

9. Prognosis

Depends upon Metastatic spread, large tumor size, and hormonal hypersecretion as well as gender, age, and histopathological high-grade, Ki67 (**Table 13**).

SEER Stage	5-year Relative Survival Rate
Localized	93%
Regional	77%
Distant	27%
All SEER stages combined	54%

Table 13.
5-year relative survival rates for pancreatic NET [8].

10. Conclusion

Pancreatic neuroendocrine tumors are a distinct group of tumors from other pancreatic malignancies. They present with vastly different spectrum of clinical features ranging from asymptomatic incidentalomas to symptoms related to hormone hypersecretion or due to mass effect. Due to rarity of these tumors and as the biological potential of these tumors remain unexplored, the management is largely consensus based and is still under a lot of research. Although surgery is the main modality of treatment but conservative management is also indicated in small non functioning tumors. Advanced pNET can be treated with chemotherapy or targeted agents. In this context, prospective studies with the creation of a large multi-center trials and an international registry are future recommendations.

Conflict of interest

The authors declare no conflict of interest.

Thanks

A special thanks to Dr. Vivck Sharma for his invaluable contribution.

Author details

Neha Sharma[1*] and Deepti Sharma[2]

1 Department of Radiation Oncology, Lady Hardinge Medical College and Associated SSK and KSC Hospital, India

2 Department of Radiation Oncology, Institute of Liver and Biliary Science, India

*Address all correspondence to: mailnehash@gmail.com

References

[1] Taal BG, Visser O. Epidemiology of neuroendocrine tumours Vol. 80, Suppl. 1, 2004. Neuroendocrinology 2004;80:104–. doi:10.1159/000081547.

[2] Massironi S, Sciola V, Peracchi M, Ciafardini C, Spampatti MP, Conte D. Neuroendocrine tumors of the gastro-entero-pancreatic system. World Journal of Gastroenterology 2008;14:5377. doi:10.3748/wjg.14.5377.

[3] Warner RR. Enteroendocrine Tumors Other Than Carcinoid: A Review of Clinically Significant Advances. Gastroenterology 2005;128:1668-84. doi:10.1053/j.gastro.2005.03.078.

[4] Yao JC, Hassan M, Phan A, Dagohoy C, Leary C, Mares JE, et al. One Hundred Years After "Carcinoid": Epidemiology of and Prognostic Factors for Neuroendocrine Tumors in 35,825 Cases in the United States. Journal of Clinical Oncology 2008;26:3063-72. doi:10.1200/jco.2007.15.4377.

[5] B. Lawrence, B. I. Gustafsson, A. Chan, B. Svejda, M. Kidd, and I. M. Modlin, "The epidemiology of gastroenteropancreatic neuroendocrine tumors," *Endocrinology and Metabolism Clinics of North America*, vol. 40, no. 1, pp. 1-18, 2011.

[6] Ehehalt F, Saeger HD, Schmidt CM, Grützmann R. Neuroendocrine Tumors of the Pancreas. The Oncologist 2009;14:456-67. doi:10.1634/theoncologist.2008-0259.

[7] Watley DC, Ly QP, Talmon G, Are C, Sasson AR. Clinical presentation and outcome of non-functional pancreatic neuroendocrine tumors in a modern cohort. Am J Surg. 2015;210(6):1192-6.

[8] Key Statistics for Pancreatic Neuroendocrine Tumor. American Cancer Society. https://www.cancer.org/cancer/pancreatic-neuroendocrine-tumor/about/key-statistics.html.

[9] Wilde RFD, Edil BH, Hruban RH, Maitra A. Well-differentiated pancreatic neuroendocrine tumors: from genetics to therapy. Nature Reviews Gastroenterology & Hepatology 2012;9:199-208. doi:10.1038/nrgastro.2012.9.

[10] Falconi M, Eriksson B, Kaltsas G, Bartsch D, Capdevila J, Caplin M, et al. ENETS Consensus Guidelines Update for the Management of Patients with Functional Pancreatic Neuroendocrine Tumors and Non-Functional Pancreatic Neuroendocrine Tumors. Neuroendocrinology 2016;103:153-71. doi:10.1159/000443171.

[11] Halfdanarson T, Rabe K, Rubin J, Petersen G. Pancreatic neuroendocrine tumors (PNETs): incidence, prognosis and recent trend toward improved survival. Annals of Oncology 2008;19:1727-33. doi:10.1093/annonc/mdn351.

[12] Rindi G Falconi M, Klersy C, Albarello L, Boninsegna L, Buchler MW, et al., TNM staging of neoplasms of the endocrine pancreas: results from a large international cohort study. J Natl Cancer Inst 2012; 104: 764-77.

[13] Ueda Y, Toyama H, Fukumoto T, Ku Y. Prognosis of Patients with Neuroendocrine Neoplasms of the Pancreas According to the World Health Organization 2017 Classification. JOP Journal of the Pancreas 2017. https://pancreas.imedpub.com/prognosis-of-patients-with-neuroendocrine-neoplasms-of-the-pancreas-according-to-the-world-health-organization-2017-classification.php?aid=21167#11.

[14] Cavalcanti MS, Gönen M, Klimstra DS. The ENETS/WHO grading system for neuroendocrine neoplasms of the gastroenteropancreatic system: a review of the current state, limitations and proposals for modifications.

Int J Endocr Oncol. 2016;3(3):203-219. doi:10.2217/ije-2016-0006

[15] Lloyd RV, Osamura RY, Klöppel G, Rosai J. WHO Classification of Tumours of Endocrine Organs 4th ed. Lyon: IARC, 2017

[16] Klöppel G, Rindi G, Perren A, Komminoth P, Klimstra DS. The ENETS and AJCC/UICC TNM classifications of the neuroendocrine tumors of the gastrointestinal tract and the pancreas: a statement. Virchows Archiv 2010;456:595-7. doi:10.1007/s00428-010-0924-6.

[17] Seydafkan S, Coppola D. Neuroendocrine Tumor Classification Systems: Staging. Neuroendocrine Tumors: Review of Pathology, Molecular and Therapeutic Advances 2016:21-30. doi:10.1007/978-1-4939-3426-3_2.

[18] Cubilla AL, Fitzgerald PJ. Cancer of the exocrine pancreas: the pathologic aspects. CA Cancer J Clin. 1985;35:2-18. doi: 10.3322/canjclin.35.1.2.

[19] Shimada N, Miwa S, Arai T, Kitagawa N, Akita S, Iinuma N, et al. Cystic mixed adenoneuroendocrine carcinoma of the pancreas: A case report. International Journal of Surgery Case Reports. 2018;52:1-4.

[20] Lee HH, Jung CK, Jung ES, Song KY, Jeon HM, Park CH. Mixed Exocrine and Endocrine Carcinoma in the Stomach: A Case Report. Journal of Gastric Cancer. 2011;11(2):122.

[21] Imaoka K, Fukuda S, Tazawa H, Kuga Y, Mochizuki T, Hirata Y, et al. A mixed adenoneuroendocrine carcinoma of the pancreas: a case report. Surgical Case Reports. 2016;2(1).

[22] Asa S. Pancreatic endocrine tumors. Modern Pathology. 2011;24(S2):S66-S77.

[23] PavlidisTE, PsarrasK, SymeonidisNG, Pavlidis ET, Sakantamis AK. Current surgical management of pancreatic endocrine tumor liver metastases. Hepatobiliary Pancreat Dis Int. 2011;10(3):243-7.

[24] Reid MD, Balci S, Saka B, Adsay NV. Neuroendocrine Tumors of the Pancreas: Current Concepts and Controversies. Endocrine Pathology 2014;25:65-79. doi:10.1007/s12022-013-9295-2.

[25] Andrew A, Kramer B, Rawdon BB. The origin of gut and pancreatic neuroendocrine (APUD) cells—the last word? The Journal of Pathology 1998;186:117-8. doi:10.1002/(sici)1096-9896(1998100)186:2<117::aid-path152>3.0.co;2-j.

[26] Jones S, Zhang X, Parsons DW, et al. Core signaling pathways in human pancreatic cancers revealed by global genomic analyses. Science. 2008;321:1801-6.

[27] Antonello D, Gobbo S, Corbo V, Sipos B, Lemoine NR, Scarpa A. Update on the molecular pathogenesis of pancreatic tumors other than common ductal adenocarcinoma. Pancreatology. 2009;9(1-2):25-33.

[28] Fasanella KE, McGrath KM, Sanders M, Brody D, Domsic R, Khalid A. Pancreatic endocrine tumor EUS-guided FNA DNA microsatellite loss and mortality. Gastrointest Endosc. 2009;69(6):1074-80.

[29] Oberg K. Genetics and molecular pathology of neuroendocrine gastrointestinal and pancreatic tumors (gastroenteropancreatic neuroendocrine tumors). Curr Opin Endocrinol Diabetes Obes. 2009;16(1):72-8.

[30] Zimmermann N, Knief J, Kacprowski T, Lazar-Karsten P, Keck T, Billmann F, et al. MicroRNA analysis of gastroenteropancreatic neuroendocrine tumors and metastases. Oncotarget. 2018;9(47):28379-90

[31] Satapathy S, Batra J, Jeet V, Thompson EW, Punyadeera C. MicroRNAs in HPV associated cancers: small players with big consequences. Expert Review of Molecular Diagnostics. 2017;17(7):711-22.

[32] Garzon R, Marcucci G, Croce CM. Targeting microRNAs in cancer: rationale, strategies and challenges. Nat Rev Drug Discov. 2010;9:775-89. doi: 10.1038/nrd3179.

[33] Calin GA, Croce CM. MicroRNA signatures in human cancers. Nature Reviews Cancer. 2006;6(11):857-66.

[34] Meiri E, Mueller WC, Rosenwald S, Zepeniuk M, Klinke E, Edmonston TB, Werner M, Lass U, Barshack I, Feinmesser M, Huszar M, Fogt F, Ashkenazi K, et al. A second-generation microRNA-based assay for diagnosing tumor tissue origin. Oncologist. 2012;17:801-12. doi: 10.1634/theoncologist.2011-0466.

[35] Thorns C, Schurmann C, Gebauer N, Wallaschofski H, Kümpers C, Bernard V, Feller AC, Keck T, Habermann JK, Begum N, Lehnert H, Brabant G. Global microRNA profiling of pancreatic neuroendocrine neoplasias. Anticancer Res. 2014;34:2249-54.

[36] Ruebel K, Leontovich AA, Stilling GA, Zhang S, Righi A, Jin L, Lloyd RV. MicroRNA expression in ileal carcinoid tumors: downregulation of microRNA-133a with tumor progression. Mod Pathol. 2010;23:367-75. doi: 10.1038/modpathol.2009.161.

[37] Pantel K, Speicher MR. The biology of circulating tumor cells. Oncogene. 2015;35(10):1216-24

[38] Hsieh JC-H, Chen G-Y, Jhou DD-W, Chou W-C, Yeh C-N, Hwang T-L, et al. The Prognostic Value of Circulating Tumor Cells in Asian Neuroendocrine Tumors. Scientific Reports. 2019;9(1).

[39] Khan MS, Tsigani T, Rashid M, Rabouhans JS, Yu D, Luong TV, et al. Circulating Tumor Cells and EpCAM Expression in Neuroendocrine Tumors. Clinical Cancer Research. 2011;17(2):337-45.

[40] Fischer C, Pape U-F, Neumann T, Detjen KM, Hilfenhaus G, Hess G, et al. Prognostic relevance of circulating PIGF levels in patients with neuroendocrine tumors. Journal of Clinical Oncology. 2012;30(15_suppl):4128

[41] L. R. McKenna and B. H. Edil, "Update on pancreatic neuroendocrine tumors," *Gland Surgery*, vol. 3, no. 4, pp. 258-275, 2014.

[42] Ro C, Chai W, Yu VE, Yu R. Pancreatic neuroendocrine tumors: biology, diagnosis,and treatment. *Chin J Cancer*. 2013;32(6):312-324. doi:10.5732/cjc.012.10295

[43] Alexakis N, Neoptolemos JP. Pancreatic neuroendocrine tumours. *Best Pract Res Clin Gastroenterol*. 2008;22(1):183-205. doi:10.1016/j.bpg.2007.10.008

[44] Ito T, Igarashi H, Jensen RT. Pancreatic neuroendocrine tumors: Clinical features, diagnosis and medical treatment: Advances. Best Practice & Research Clinical Gastroenterology. 2012;26(6):737-53.

[45] Zhuo F. Insulinoma [Internet]. StatPearls [Internet]. U.S. National Library of Medicine; 2019. Available from: https://www.ncbi.nlm.nih.gov/books/NBK544299/

[46] Feliberti E. Gastrinoma [Internet]. Endotext [Internet]. U.S. National Library of Medicine; 2017. Available from:https://www.ncbi.nlm.nih.gov/books/NBK279075/

[47] Sandhu S. Glucagonoma Syndrome [Internet]. StatPearls [Internet]. U.S. National Library of Medicine; 2020.

Available from: https://www. ncbi.nlm. nih.gov/books/NBK519500/

[48] Sandhu S. ViPoma [Internet]. StatPearls [Internet]. U.S. National Library of Medicine; 2019. Available from: https://www.ncbi.nlm.nih.gov/books/NBK507698/

[49] Williamson JM, Thorn CC, Spalding D, Williamson RC. Pancreatic and peripancreatic somatostatinomas. *Ann R Coll Surg Engl*. 2011;93(5):356-360. doi:10.1308/003588411X582681

[50] Park YS. Less Common Types of Pancreatic Neuroendocrine Tumors. Neuroendocrine Tumours. 2015;:271-4.

[51] Lee DW, Kim MK, Kim HG. Diagnosis of Pancreatic Neuroendocrine Tumors. Clinical Endoscopy. 2017; 50(6):537-45.

[52] Viudez A, De Jesus-Acosta A, Carbalho FL, Vera R, Martin-Algarra S, Ramirez N. Pancreatic neuroendocrine tumors: challenges in an underestimated disease. Crit Rev Oncol Hematol. 2016;101:193-206.

[53] Jun E, Kim SC, Song KB, et al. Diagnostic value of chromogranin A in pancreatic neuroendocrine tumors depends on tumor size: A prospective observational study from a single institute. *Surgery*. 2017;162(1):120-130. doi:10.1016/j.surg.2017.01.019

[54] Ramage JK. Guidelines for the management of gastroenteropancreatic neuroendocrine (including carcinoid) tumours. Gut 2005;54:iv1–iv16. doi:10.1136/gut.2004.053314.

[55] Khashab MA, Yong E, Lennon AM, et al. EUS is still superior to multidetector computerized tomography for detection of pancreatic neuroendocrine tumors. Gastrointest Endosc. 2011;73:691-6.

[56] Reidy-Lagunes DL, Gollub MJ, Saltz LB. Addition of Octreotide Functional Imaging to Cross-Sectional Computed Tomography or Magnetic Resonance Imaging for the Detection of Neuroendocrine Tumors: Added Value or an Anachronism? Journal of Clinical Oncology 2011;29. doi:10.1200/jco.2010.32.8559.

[57] James PD, Tsolakis AV, Zhang M, Belletrutti PJ, Mohamed R, Roberts DJ, et al. Incremental benefit of preoperative EUS for the detection of pancreatic neuroendocrine tumors: a meta-analysis. Gastrointestinal Endoscopy 2015;81. doi:10.1016/j.gie.2014.12.031.

[58] Zimmer T, Stolzel U, Bader M, Koppenhagen K, Hamm B, Buhr H, et al. Endoscopic ultrasonography and somatostatin receptor scintigraphy in the preoperative localisation of insulinomas and gastrinomas. Gut 1996;39:562-8. doi:10.1136/gut.39.4.562.

[59] Westlin J-E, Janson ET, Arnberg H, Ahlström H, Öberg K, Nilsson S. Somatostatin Receptor Scintigraphy of Carcinoid Tumours Using the [111In-Dtpa-D-Phe1]-Octreotide. Acta Oncologica 1993;32:783-6. doi:10.3109/02841869309096136.

[60] PapottiM, BongiovanniM, VolanteM, et al. Expression of somatostatin receptor types 1-5 in 81 cases of gastrointestinal and pancreatic endocrine tumors. A correlative immunohistochemical and reverse-transcriptase polymerase chain reaction analysis. Virchows Arch. 2002;440:461-75

[61] Jabiev AA, Lew JI. In Reply: Surgeon-Performed Ultrasound and Prediction of Differentiated Thyroid Cancer. Annals of Surgical Oncology 2010;18:301–. doi:10.1245/s10434-010-1312-9.

[62] Raj N, Reidy-Lagunes D. The Role of 68Ga-DOTATATE Positron Emission Tomography/Computed Tomography in Well-Differentiated Neuroendocrine Tumors. Pancreas 2018;47:1-5. Doi: 10.1097/MPA.0000000000000949

[63] Heitz PU KP, Perren A, Klimstra D, et al. Tumors of the endocrine pancreas. In: DeLellis RA LR, Heitz PU, Eng C, eds. Pathology and Genetics of Tumours of Endocrine Organs. Lyon: France IARC Press, 2004:175-208.

[64] Sopha S. Neuroendocrine neoplasms - general. PathologyOutlines.com website. http://www.pathologyoutlines.com/topic/pancreaspen.html. Accessed May 5th, 2020.

[65] Well Differentiated Pancreatic Neuroendocrine Tumor / Islet Cell Tumor [Internet]. Differential Diagnosis - Well Differentiated Pancreatic Endocrine Neoplasm (Islet Cell Tumor) - Surgical Pathology Criteria - Stanford University School of Medicine. Available from: http://surgpathcriteria.stanford.edu/pancreas/well-differentiated-pancreatic-neuroendocrine-neoplasm-tumor-islet-cell/differentialdiagnosis.html#t5

[66] Glucagonoma Differential Diagnoses. 2020. Available from:https://emedicine.medscape.com/article/118899-differential

[67] Teh SH, Deveney C, Sheppard BC. Aggressive pancreatic resection for primary pancreatic neuroendocrine tumor: is it justifiable? Am J Surg. 2007;193:610-3.

[68] Hashim YM, Trinkaus KM, Linehan DC, Strasberg SS, Fields RC, Cao D, et al. Regional lymphadenectomy is indicated in the surgical treatment of pancreatic neuroendocrine tumors (PNETs). Ann Surg. 2014;259(2):197-203.

[69] Pathak S, Dash I, Taylor MR et al The surgical management of neuroendocrine tumour hepatic metastases. Eur. J. Surg. Oncol. 39, 224-228 (2013).

[70] Pancreatic Neuroendocrine Tumors in the 21st Century –An Update [Internet]. Clinicsinsurgery.com. 2020 [cited 9 May 2020]. Available from: http://www.clinicsinsurgery.com/full-text/cis-v2-id1662.php

[71] V. Sallinen, T. Y. S. le Large, S. Galeev et al., "Surveillance strategy for small asymptomatic non-functional pancreatic neuroendocrine tumors – a systematic review and meta-analysis," HPB: The Official Journal of the International Hepato Pancreato Biliary Association, vol. 19, no. 4, pp. 310-320, 2017.

[72] J. Chabot, "Editorial: pancreatic neuroendocrine tumors: primum non nocere," *Surgery*, vol. 159, no. 1, pp. 348-349, 2016.

[73] F. J. Hüttner, J. Koessler-Ebs, T. Hackert, A. Ulrich, M. W. Büchler, and M. K. Diener, "Meta-analysis of surgical outcome after enucleation *versus* standard resection for pancreatic neoplasms," *British Journal of Surgery*, vol. 102, no. 9, pp. 1026-1036, 2015.

[74] S. Gaujoux, S. Partelli, F. Maire et al., "Observational study of natural history of small sporadic nonfunctioning pancreatic neuroendocrine tumors," *The Journal of Clinical Endocrinology and Metabolism*, vol. 98, no. 12, pp. 4784-4789, 2013.

[75] L. C. Lee, C. S. Grant, D. R. Salomao et al., "Small, nonfunctioning, asymptomatic pancreatic neuroendocrine tumors (PNETs): role for nonoperative management," *Surgery*, vol. 152, no. 6, pp. 965-974, 2012.

[76] E. Sadot, D. L. Reidy-Lagunes, L. H. Tang et al., "Observation versus resection for small asymptomatic pancreatic neuroendocrine tumors: a matched case-control study," *Annals of Surgical Oncology*, vol. 23, no. 4, pp. 1361-1370, 2016.

[77] Rosenberg AM, Friedmann P, Rivero JD, Libutti SK, Laird AM. Resection versus expectant management of small incidentally discovered nonfunctional pancreatic

neuroendocrine tumors. Surgery 2016;159:302-10. doi:10.1016/j.surg.2015.10.013.

[78] Regenet N, Carrere N, Boulanger G, Calan LD, Humeau M, Arnault V, et al. Is the 2-cm size cutoff relevant for small nonfunctioning pancreatic neuroendocrine tumors: A French multicenter study. Surgery 2016;159:901-7. doi:10.1016/j.surg.2015.10.003.

[79] Zhang, I.Y., Zhao, J., Fernandez-del Castillo, C. *et al.* Operative Versus Nonoperative Management of Nonfunctioning Pancreatic Neuroendocrine Tumors. *J Gastrointest Surg* 20, 277-283 (2016). https://doi.org/10.1007/s11605-015-3043-5

[80] Shah MH, Goldner WS, Halfdanarson TR, Bergsland E, Berlin JD, Halperin D, et al. NCCN Guidelines Insights: Neuroendocrine and Adrenal Tumors, Version 2.2018. Journal of the National Comprehensive Cancer Network 2018;16:693-702. doi:10.6004/jnccn.2018.0056.

[81] Cherenfant J, Stocker SJ, Gage MK, Du H, Thurow TA, Odeleye M, et al. Predicting aggressive behavior in nonfunctioning pancreatic neuroendocrine tumors. Surgery 2013;154:785-93. doi:10.1016/j.surg.2013.07.004

[82] Panzuto F, Boninsegna L, Fazio N, Campana D, Brizzi MP, Capurso G, et al. Metastatic and Locally Advanced Pancreatic Endocrine Carcinomas: Analysis of Factors Associated With Disease Progression. Journal of Clinical Oncology 2011;29:2372-7. doi:10.1200/jco.2010.33.0688.

[83] Eriksson B. New drugs in neuroendocrine tumors: rising of new therapeutic philosophies? Current Opinion in Oncology 2010;22:381-6. doi:10.1097/cco.0b013e32833adee2.

[84] Rinke A, Müller H-H, Schade-Brittinger C, Klose K-J, Barth P, Wied M, et al. Placebo-Controlled, Double-Blind, Prospective, Randomized Study on the Effect of Octreotide LAR in the Control of Tumor Growth in Patients With Metastatic Neuroendocrine Midgut Tumors: A Report From the PROMID Study Group. Journal of Clinical Oncology 2009;27:4656-63. doi:10.1200/jco.2009.22.8510.

[85] Caplin ME, Pavel M, Ćwikła JB, Phan AT, Raderer M, Sedláčková E, et al. LanreotideinMetastaticEnteropancreatic Neuroendocrine Tumors. New England Journal of Medicine 2014;371:224-33. doi:10.1056/nejmoa1316158.

[86] Wolin E, Jarzab B, Eriksson B, Walter T, Toumpanakis C, Morse MA, et al. Phase III study of pasireotide long-acting release in patients with metastatic neuroendocrine tumors and carcinoid symptoms refractory to available somatostatin analogues. Drug Design, Development and Therapy 2015:5075. doi:10.2147/dddt.s84177.

[87] Chan D.L., Ferone D., Albertelli M., Pavlakis N., Segelov E., Singh S. Escalated-dose somatostatin analogues for antiproliferative effect in GEPNETS: A systematic review. Endocrine. 2017;57:366-375. doi: 10.1007/s12020-017-1360-z.

[88] Mohamed A., Blanchard M.P., Albertelli M., Barbieri F., Brue T., Niccoli P., Delpero J.R., Monges G., Garcia S., Ferone D., et al. Pasireotide and octreotide antiproliferative effects and sst2 trafficking in human pancreatic neuroendocrine tumor cultures. Endocr. Relat. Cancer. 2014;21:691-704. doi: 10.1530/ERC-14-0086.

[89] Cives M., Kunz P.L., Morse B., Coppola D., Schell M.J., Campos T., Nguyen P.T., Nandoskar P., Khandelwal V., Strosberg J.R. Phase II clinical trial of pasireotide long-acting repeatable in patients with metastatic neuroendocrine

tumors. Endocr. Relat. Cancer. 2015;22:1-9. doi: 10.1530/ERC-14-0360.

[90] Kulke M.H., Ruszniewski P., Van Cutsem E., Lombard-Bohas C., Valle J.W., De Herder W.W., Pavel M., Degtyarev E., Brase J.C., Bubuteishvili-Pacaud L., et al. A randomized, open-label, phase 2 study of everolimus in combination with pasireotide LAR or everolimus alone in advanced, well-differentiated, progressive pancreatic neuroendocrine tumors: COOPERATE-2 trial. Ann. Oncol. 2017;28:1309-1315. doi: 10.1093/annonc/mdx078.

[91] 1. Kulke M, Lenz H, Meropol N, Posey J, Ryan D, Picus J et al. Activity of Sunitinib in Patients With Advanced Neuroendocrine Tumors. Journal of Clinical Oncology. 2008;26(20):3403-3410.

[92] 2. Raymond E, Dahan L, Raoul J, Bang Y, Borbath I, Lombard-Bohas C et al. Sunitinib Malate for the Treatment of Pancreatic Neuroendocrine Tumors. New England Journal of Medicine. 2011;364(6):501-513.

[93] Yao J, Lombard-Bohas C, Baudin E, Kvols L, Rougier P, Ruszniewski P et al. Daily Oral Everolimus Activity in Patients With Metastatic Pancreatic Neuroendocrine Tumors After Failure of Cytotoxic Chemotherapy: A Phase II Trial. Journal of Clinical Oncology. 2010;28(1):69-76.

[94] Yao J, Phan A, Chang D, Wolff R, Hess K, Gupta S et al. Efficacy of RAD001 (Everolimus) and Octreotide LAR in Advanced Low- to Intermediate-Grade Neuroendocrine Tumors: Results of a Phase II Study. Journal of Clinical Oncology. 2008;26(26):4311-4318.

[95] Yao J, Shah M, Ito T, Bohas C, Wolin E, Van Cutsem E et al. Everolimus for Advanced Pancreatic Neuroendocrine Tumors. New England Journal of Medicine. 2011;364(6):514-523.

[96] Duran I, Kortmansky J, Singh D, Hirte H, Kocha W, Goss G et al. A phase II clinical and pharmacodynamic study of temsirolimus in advanced neuroendocrine carcinomas. British Journal of Cancer. 2006;95(9):1148-1

[97] Hobday TJ, Rubin J, Holen K, et al. MC044h, a phase II trial of sorafenib in patients (pts) with metastatic neuroendocrine tumors (NET): A Phase II Consortium (P2C) study. J Clin Oncol. 2007;25:18s. (Suppl; abstr 4504) [

[98] Phan AT, Yao JC, Fogelman DR, et al. A prospective, multi-institutional phase II study of GW786034 (pazopanib) and depot octreotide (sandostatin LAR) in advanced low-grade neuroendocrine carcinoma (LGNEC) J Clin Oncol. 2010;28:15s. (Suppl; abstr 4001)

[99] Broder, L. E. & Carter, S. K. Pancreatic islet cell carcinoma. II. Results of therapy with streptozotocin in 52 patients. Ann. Intern. Med. 79, 108-118 (1973)

[100] Kulke, M. H. et al. Phase II study of temozolomide and thalidomide in patients with metastatic neuroendocrine tumors. J. Clin. Oncol. 24, 401-406 (2006)

[101] Moertel C, Hanley J, Johnson L. Streptozocin Alone Compared with Streptozocin plus Fluorouracil in the Treatment of Advanced Islet-Cell Carcinoma. New England Journal of Medicine. 1980;303(21):1189-1194.

[102] Moertel C, Lefkopoulo M, Lipsitz S, Hahn R, Klaassen D. Streptozocin–Doxorubicin, Streptozocin–Fluorouracil, or Chlorozotocin in the Treatment of Advanced Islet-Cell Carcinoma. New England Journal of Medicine. 1992;326(8):519-523.

[103] Moertel C, Kvols L, O'Connell M, Rubin J. Treatment of neuroendocrine carcinomas with combined etoposide and cisplatin. Evidence of major

therapeutic activity in the anaplastic variants of these neoplasms. Cancer. 1991;68(2):227-232.

[104] Turner N, Strauss S, Sarker D, Gillmore R, Kirkwood A, Hackshaw A et al. Chemotherapy with 5-fluorouracil, cisplatin and streptozocin for neuroendocrine tumours. British Journal of Cancer. 2010;102(7):1106-1112.

[105] Ramanathan R, Cnaan A, Hahn R, Carbone P, Haller D. Phase II trial of dacarbazine (DTIC) in advanced pancreatic islet cell carcinoma. Study of the Eastern Cooperative Oncology Group-E6282. Annals of Oncology. 2001;12(8):1139-1143.

[106] Bajetta E, Catena L, Procopio G, De Dosso S, Bichisao E, Ferrari L et al. Are capecitabine and oxaliplatin (XELOX) suitable treatments for progressing low-grade and high-grade neuroendocrine tumours?. Cancer Chemotherapy and Pharmacology. 2006;59(5):637-642.

[107] Kulke M, Stuart K, Enzinger P, Ryan D, Clark J, Muzikansky A et al. Phase II Study of Temozolomide and Thalidomide in Patients With Metastatic Neuroendocrine Tumors. Journal of Clinical Oncology. 2006;24(3):401-406.

[108] Chan JA, Stuart K, Earle CC, et al. Prospective study of bevacizumab plus temozolomide in patients with advanced neuroendocrine tumors. *J Clin Oncol*. 2012;30(24):2963-2968. doi:10.1200/JCO.2011.40.3147

[109] Chan J, Blaszkowsky L, Stuart K, Zhu A, Allen J, Wadlow R et al. A prospective, phase 1/2 study of everolimus and temozolomide in patients with advanced pancreatic neuroendocrine tumor. Cancer. 2013;119(17):3212-3218.

[110] Ducreux M, Dahan L, Smith D, O'Toole D, Lepère C, Dromain C et al. Bevacizumab combined with 5-FU/streptozocin in patients with progressive metastatic well-differentiated pancreatic endocrine tumours (BETTER trial) – A phase II non-randomised trial. European Journal of Cancer. 2014;50(18):3098-3106.

[111] Fani M, Maecke H, Okarvi S. Radiolabeled Peptides: Valuable Tools for the Detection and Treatment of Cancer. Theranostics. 2012;2(5):481-501.

[112] Van Essen M, Krenning E, De Jong M, Valkema R, Kwekkeboom D. Peptide Receptor Radionuclide Therapy with radiolabelled somatostatin analogues in patients with somatostatin receptor positive tumours. Acta Oncologica. 2007;46(6):723-734.

[113] Imhof A, Brunner P, Marincek N, Briel M, Schindler C, Rasch H, et al. Response, survival, and long-term toxicity after therapy with the radiolabeled somatostatin analogue [90Y-DOTA]-TOC in metastasized neuroendocrine cancers. J Clin Oncol. 2011;29(17):2416.

[114] Valkema R., Pauwels S., Kvols L.K., Barone R., Jamar F., Bakker W.H., Kwekkeboom D.J., Bouterfa H., Krenning E.P. Survival and Response after Peptide Receptor Radionuclide Therapy with [90Y-DOTA0, Tyr3] Octreotide in Patients with Advanced Gastroenteropancreatic Neuroendocrine Tumors. Elsevier; Amsterdam, The Netherlands: 2006. pp. 147-156. Seminars in Nuclear Medicine.

[115] Kwekkeboom D.J., de Herder W.W., Kam B.L., van Eijck C.H., van Essen M., Kooij P.P., Feelders R.A., van Aken M.O., Krenning E.P. Treatment with the radiolabeled somatostatin analog [177 Lu-DOTA 0, Tyr3] octreotate: Toxicity, efficacy, and survival. J. Clin. Oncol. 2008;26:2124-2130. doi: 10.1200/JCO.2007.15.2553.

[116] Bushnell D.L., Jr., O'Dorisio T.M., O'Dorisio M.S., Menda Y., Hicks R.J., Van CutsemE.,BaulieuJ.-L.,Borson-ChazotF., Anthony L., Benson A.B. 90Y-edotreotide

for metastatic carcinoid refractory to octreotide. J. Clin. Oncol. 2010;28:1652-1659. doi: 10.1200/JCO.2009.22.8585.

[117] Cwikla J., Sankowski A., Seklecka N., Buscombe J., Nasierowska-Guttmejer A., Jeziorski K., Mikolajczak R., Pawlak D., Stepien K., Walecki J. Efficacy of radionuclide treatment DOTATATE Y-90 in patients with progressive metastatic gastroenteropancreatic neuroendocrine carcinomas (GEP-NETs): A phase II study. Ann. Oncol. 2009;21:787-794. doi: 10.1093/annonc/mdp372.

[118] Pfeifer A.K., Gregersen T., Grønbæk H., Hansen C.P., Müller-Brand J., Bruun K.H., Krogh K., Kjær A., Knigge U. Peptide receptor radionuclide therapy with 90Y-DOTATOC and 177Lu-DOTATOC in advanced neuroendocrine tumors: Results from a Danish cohort treated in Switzerland. Neuroendocrinology. 2011;93:189-196. doi: 10.1159/000324096.

[119] Bodei L., Cremonesi M., Grana C.M., Fazio N., Iodice S., Baio S.M., Bartolomei M., Lombardo D., Ferrari M.E., Sansovini M., et al. Peptide receptor radionuclide therapy with 177Lu-DOTATATE: The IEO phase I-II study. Eur. J. Nucl. Med. Mol. Imaging. 2011;38:2125-2135. doi: 10.1007/s00259-011-1902-1

[120] Ezziddin S., Attassi M., Yong-Hing C.J., Ahmadzadehfar H., Willinek W., Grünwald F., Guhlke S., Biersack H.-J., Sabet A. Predictors of long-term outcome in patients with well-differentiated gastroenteropancreatic neuroendocrine tumors after peptide receptor radionuclide therapy with 177Lu-octreotate. J. Nucl. Med. 2014;55:183-190. doi: 10.2967/jnumed.113.125336.

[121] Nwosu AC, Jones L, Vora J, Poston GJ, Vinjamuri S, Pritchard DM. Assessment of the efficacy and toxicity of (131)I-metaiodobenzylguanidine therapy for metastatic neuroendocrine tumours. Br J Cancer. 2008;98(6):1053.